THIS KETO DIET

Journal Belongs To:

_____

KETO BEFORE & After

WEIGHT	WEIGHT
BMI	BMI
BODY FAT	BODY FAT
MUSCLE	MUSCLE
CHEST	CHEST
WAIST	WAIST
HIPS	HIPS
THIGHS	THIGHS
CALF	CALF
BICEP	BICEP
OTHER :	OTHER :
OTHER :	OTHER :

WEIGHT LOSS *Tracker*

MONTHLY GOAL

DATE:

	BUST			
	WAIST			
	HIPS			
	BICEP			
	THIGH			
	CALF			
	WEIGHT			
TOTAL WEIGHT LOSS >>				

MONTHLY PROGRESS *Tracker*

JAN FEB MAR APR MAY JUN JUL AUG SEP OCT NOV DEC

MON	TUE	WED	THU	FRI	SAT	SUN

WEIGHT LOSS MILESTONE TRACKER

CHEAT DAY TRACKER

WEEKLY DIET SUCCESS TRACKER & NOTES

Keto 15 Task Challenge

1

CREATE A KETO JOURNAL AND DOCUMENT YOUR PROGRESS

COMPLETED

2

CHOOSE 7 KETO FRIENDLY RECIPES TO TRY

COMPLETED

3

CREATE A WEEKLY MEAL PLANNER

COMPLETED

4

LOG EVERYTHING YOU EAT IN A WEIGHT LOSS APP

COMPLETED

5

PURCHASE A FOOD SCALE AND SPIRALIZER

COMPLETED

6

TRY BULLET PROOF COFFEE

COMPLETED

7

WEIGH YOURSELF EVERY WEEK

COMPLETED

8

GO ALCOHOL FREE FOR ONE WEEK

COMPLETED

9

TRY A 12-HOUR INTERMITTENT FAST

COMPLETED

10

CHECK AND LOG YOUR BODY MEASUREMENTS

COMPLETED

11

LIST ALL THE REASONS WHY KETO WILL WORK FOR YOU

COMPLETED

12

LEARN TO MAKE FAT BOMBS

COMPLETED

13

MONITOR YOUR WATER INTAKE

COMPLETED

14

INCREASE YOUR HEALTHY FAT INTAKE

COMPLETED

15

TEST KETONE LEVELS USING STRIPS

COMPLETED

Ketogenic Foods

MEATS

- Beef
- Sausage
- Bacon
- Lamb
- Pork
- Veal
- Chicken/Turkey
- Eggs

VEGGIES

- Avocado
- Asparagus
- Argula
- Broccoli
- Cauliflower
- Brussel Sprouts
- Cabbage
- Celery

VEGGIES

- Cucumber
- Chards
- Bell Peppers
- Green Beans
- Collards
- Mushrooms
- Spinach
- Olives

FRUITS

- Blackberries
- Cranberries
- Blueberries
- Lemon
- Lime
- Raspberries
- Strawberries
- Plantains (paleo)

DAIRY

- Cheese (all kinds)
- Sour Cream
- Cream Cheese
- Heavy Cream
- Greek Yogurt
- Almond Milk
- Cashew Milk
- Coconut Cream

CONDIMENTS

- Balsamic Vinegar
- Beef/Chicken Broth
- Bonito Flakes
- Tartar Sauce (keto)
- Dijon Mustard
- Mayo
- Low Sugar Ketchup
- Pickles

OILS & FATS

- Avocado Oil
- Butter
- Coconut Butter
- Duck Fat
- Lard/Ghee
- Nut Oils
- Olive Oil
- Pork Rinds

HERBS & SPICES

- Garlic
- Salt & Pepper
- Oregano
- Paprika
- Cumin
- Chili Pepper
- Basil
- Ginger

BAKING

- Almond Flour
- Almond Meal
- Cashew Flour
- Oat Fiber
- Psyllium Husk
- Whey Protein
- Flax meal
- Hazelnut Flour

FISH/SEAFOOD

- Anchovy
- Haddock / Cod
- Halibut
- Crab/Lobster
- Mackerel
- Salmon
- Tuna
- Red Snapper

DRINKS

- Diet Soda (moderation)
- Coffee
- Tea
- Gatorade Zero
- Protein Shake
- Club Soda
- Broth
- Coconut Water

MISC.

- Canned Tuna
- Pesto
- Soy Sauce
- Aioli
- Béarnaise
- Vinaigrette
- Hot Sauce
- Guacamole

NOTES:

Yearly Keto Day Tracker

JAN FEB MAR APR MAY JUN JUL AUG SEP OCT NOV DEC

1
2
3
4
5
6
7
8
9
10
11
12
13
14
15
16
17
18
19
20
21
22
23
24
25
26
27
28
29
30
31

COLOR IN THE DAYS THAT YOU WERE IN KETOSIS TO KEEP TRACK OF YOUR WEIGHT LOSS PROGRESS!

NOTES & REFLECTIONS:

TOTAL DAYS IN KETOSIS:

MONTH BY MONTH *Tracker*

MONTHLY WEIGHT LOSS TRACKER

JANUARY	JULY

FEBRUARY	AUGUST

MARCH	SEPTEMBER

APRIL	OCTOBER

MAY	NOVEMBER

JUNE	DECEMBER

MILESTONES	NOTES & REFLECTIONS

WEIGHT LOSS *Start Date*

Outline your most important fitness goals

Describe how you see yourself in six months

DATE	KETO WEIGHT LOSS ACTION PLAN		PERSONAL MILESTONES

WEIGHT LOSS *Journal*

MONDAY

TUESDAY

WEDNESDAY

THURSDAY

FRIDAY

SATURDAY

SUNDAY

WEEK OF:

DATE	WEIGHT LOSS ACTION PLAN

NOTES

MY WEIGHT LOSS *Routine*

WEIGHT LOSS SUCCESS: HABIT & ROUTINE TRACKER

DRINK LOTS OF WATER TODAY	TRACK TOTAL CARB INTAKE

COMPLETE TOP 3 GOALS OF THE DAY

1

2

3

PLAN MY MEALS FOR THE DAY:

BREAKFAST	LUNCH	DINNER

DAILY TRACKER & TO DO LIST	ACCOMPLISHMENTS

NOTES

MY KETO *Routine*

Morning	My Weight Loss Routine	m t w t f s s

Mid Day	My Weight Loss Routine	m t w t f s s

Evening	My Weight Loss Routine	m t w t f s s

Night	My Weight Loss Routine	m t w t f s s

WEEKLY *Fasting Tracker*

Week Of: _____

MONDAY

Goal	12	1	2	3	4	5	6	7	8	9	10	11	12	1	2	3	4	5	6	7	8	9	10	11
Actual	12	1	2	3	4	5	6	7	8	9	10	11	12	1	2	3	4	5	6	7	8	9	10	11

TUESDAY

Goal	12	1	2	3	4	5	6	7	8	9	10	11	12	1	2	3	4	5	6	7	8	9	10	11
Actual	12	1	2	3	4	5	6	7	8	9	10	11	12	1	2	3	4	5	6	7	8	9	10	11

WEDNESDAY

Goal	12	1	2	3	4	5	6	7	8	9	10	11	12	1	2	3	4	5	6	7	8	9	10	11
Actual	12	1	2	3	4	5	6	7	8	9	10	11	12	1	2	3	4	5	6	7	8	9	10	11

THURSDAY

Goal	12	1	2	3	4	5	6	7	8	9	10	11	12	1	2	3	4	5	6	7	8	9	10	11
Actual	12	1	2	3	4	5	6	7	8	9	10	11	12	1	2	3	4	5	6	7	8	9	10	11

FRIDAY

Goal	12	1	2	3	4	5	6	7	8	9	10	11	12	1	2	3	4	5	6	7	8	9	10	11
Actual	12	1	2	3	4	5	6	7	8	9	10	11	12	1	2	3	4	5	6	7	8	9	10	11

SATURDAY

Goal	12	1	2	3	4	5	6	7	8	9	10	11	12	1	2	3	4	5	6	7	8	9	10	11
Actual	12	1	2	3	4	5	6	7	8	9	10	11	12	1	2	3	4	5	6	7	8	9	10	11

SUNDAY

Goal	12	1	2	3	4	5	6	7	8	9	10	11	12	1	2	3	4	5	6	7	8	9	10	11
Actual	12	1	2	3	4	5	6	7	8	9	10	11	12	1	2	3	4	5	6	7	8	9	10	11

WEEKLY *Progress*

Monday

Tuesday

Wednesday

Thursday

Friday

Saturday

Sunday

Notes

KETO *Meal* LOG BOOK

	BREAKFAST	LUNCH	DINNER	SNACKS
MONDAY				
TUESDAY				
WEDNESDAY				
THURSDAY				
FRIDAY				
SATURDAY				
SUNDAY				

MY PROGRESS *Tracker*

SLEEP TRACKER:

DATE _____

| RISE: | | BEDTIME: | | SLEEP (HRS): |

NOTES FOR THE DAY

_____

_____

_____

EXERCISE / WORKOUT ROUTINE

IN A STATE OF KETOSIS?

YES   NO   UNSURE

WATER INTAKE TRACKER

DAILY ENERGY LEVEL		
HIGH	**MEDIUM**	**LOW**

BREAKFAST

FAT: CARBS: PROTEIN: CALORIES:

LUNCH

FAT: CARBS: PROTEIN: CALORIES:

DINNER

FAT: CARBS: PROTEIN: CALORIES:

SNACKS

FAT: CARBS: PROTEIN: CALORIES:

TOP 6 PRIORITIES OF THE DAY

_____

_____

_____

END OF THE DAY TOTAL OVERVIEW

CARBS	FAT	PROTEIN	CALORIES

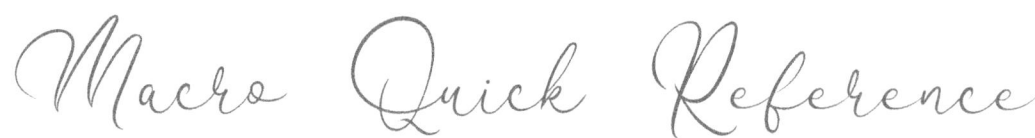

Macro Quick Reference

MACRO TRACKER

QTY	TYPE	PROTEIN	FAT	CARBS	CALS	NOTES

INTERMITTENT *Fasting Log*

WEEK OF:

	START TIME	END TIME	TOTAL FAST HRS
M	:	:	:
T	:	:	:
W	:	:	:
T	:	:	:
F	:	:	:
S	:	:	:
S	:	:	:

WEEK OF:

	START TIME	END TIME	TOTAL FAST HRS
M	:	:	:
T	:	:	:
W	:	:	:
T	:	:	:
F	:	:	:
S	:	:	:
S	:	:	:

WEEK OF:

	START TIME	END TIME	TOTAL FAST HRS
M	:	:	:
T	:	:	:
W	:	:	:
T	:	:	:
F	:	:	:
S	:	:	:
S	:	:	:

WEEK OF:

	START TIME	END TIME	TOTAL FAST HRS
M	:	:	:
T	:	:	:
W	:	:	:
T	:	:	:
F	:	:	:
S	:	:	:
S	:	:	:

WEEK OF:

	START TIME	END TIME	TOTAL FAST HRS
M	:	:	:
T	:	:	:
W	:	:	:
T	:	:	:
F	:	:	:
S	:	:	:
S	:	:	:

WEEK OF:

	START TIME	END TIME	TOTAL FAST HRS
M	:	:	:
T	:	:	:
W	:	:	:
T	:	:	:
F	:	:	:
S	:	:	:
S	:	:	:

MILESTONES & ACCOMPLISHMENTS

NOTES & REFLECTIONS

GOALS & *Accomplishments*

Month | JAN FEB MAR APR MAY JUN JUL AUG SEP OCT NOV DEC

THIS MONTH'S **GOALS**

ACTION PLAN   M T W T F S S

NOTES:

WEEKLY GOALS

M

T

W

T

F

S

S

THOUGHTS

MEALS:	BREAKFAST	LUNCH	DINNER	SNACKS
M				
T				
W				
T				
F				
S				
S				

Low Carb Grocery Ideas

FRESH PRODUCE

☐	Asparagus	☐	Cauliflower	☐	Onions
☐	Avocado	☐	Celery	☐	Radishes
☐	Bell Peppers	☐	Cucumber	☐	Salad Mix
☐	Berries	☐	Eggplant	☐	Squash
☐	Broccoli	☐	Fennel	☐	Tomatoes
☐	Brussel Sprouts	☐	Garlic	☐	Bok Choi
☐	Cabbage	☐	Green Beans	☐	Chives
☐	Carrots	☐	Mushrooms	☐	Spinach

MEAT AND SEAFOOD

☐	Bacon	☐	Lamb	☐	Fish
☐	Beef	☐	Pork	☐	Crab
☐	Bison	☐	Rotisserie Chicken	☐	Lobster
☐	Chicken	☐	Sausage	☐	Scallops
☐	Deli meat	☐	Turkey	☐	Shrimp
☐	Ground Beef / Ground Turkey	☐	Oyster	☐	Mussels

DAIRY PRODUCTS

☐	Butter	☐	Eggs	☐	Sour Cream
☐	Cheese	☐	Greek Yogurt, full fat	☐	Ghee
☐	Cream Cheese	☐	Heavy Whipping Cream	☐	Mayo

PANTRY ITEMS

☐	Avocado oil	☐	Tea/Coffee	☐	Moon Cheese
☐	Beef Jerky	☐	Pork Rinds	☐	Low Carb Protein Bars
☐	Bone Broth	☐	Mayonnaise	☐	All Natural Peanut Butter
☐	Tuna, Salmon (canned)	☐	Low Carb Salad Dressing	☐	Stevia
☐	Coconut Butter	☐	Olive oil, extra virgin	☐	Almonds
☐	Coconut Oil	☐	Olives	☐	Spices
☐	Almond Milk	☐	Sweeteners	☐	Almond Flour

FROZEN / OTHER

☐		☐		☐	
☐		☐		☐	
☐		☐		☐	
☐		☐		☐	

Low Carb Shopping List

FRESH PRODUCE

MEAT AND SEAFOOD

DAIRY PRODUCTS

PANTRY ITEMS

FROZEN / OTHER

Keto Friendly Foods

KETO FRIENDLY FOODS	NET CARBS	PROTEINS	FAT

FOODS TO EAT IN MODERATION	NET CARBS	PROTEINS	FAT

STAYING *On Track*

MY WEIGHT LOSS DIARY:

WATER TRACKER

LOW CARB SNACKS

NOTES & REMINDERS

DOODLE MY MOOD

BREAKFAST IDEAS

LUNCH IDEAS

DINNER IDEAS

STAYING *On Track*

MY WEIGHT LOSS DIARY:

_____

_____

_____

_____

WATER TRACKER

○ ○ ○ ○ ○ ○ ○

LOW CARB SNACKS

NOTES & REMINDERS

_____

_____

_____

_____

_____

_____

_____

_____

_____

DOODLE MY MOOD

BREAKFAST IDEAS

LUNCH IDEAS

DINNER IDEAS

STAYING *On Track*

MY WEIGHT LOSS DIARY:

WATER TRACKER

LOW CARB SNACKS

NOTES & REMINDERS

DOODLE MY MOOD

BREAKFAST IDEAS

LUNCH IDEAS

DINNER IDEAS

STAYING *On Track*

MY WEIGHT LOSS DIARY:

_____

_____

_____

_____

WATER TRACKER

ⵔ ⵔ ⵔ ⵔ ⵔ ⵔ ⵔ ⵔ

LOW CARB SNACKS

NOTES & REMINDERS

_____

_____

_____

_____

_____

_____

_____

_____

_____

_____

DOODLE MY MOOD

BREAKFAST IDEAS

LUNCH IDEAS

DINNER IDEAS

STAYING *On Track*

MY WEIGHT LOSS DIARY:

WATER TRACKER

LOW CARB SNACKS

NOTES & REMINDERS

DOODLE MY MOOD

BREAKFAST IDEAS

LUNCH IDEAS

DINNER IDEAS

STAYING *On Track*

MY WEIGHT LOSS DIARY:

_____

_____

_____

_____

WATER TRACKER

NOTES & REMINDERS

DOODLE MY MOOD

LOW CARB SNACKS

BREAKFAST IDEAS

LUNCH IDEAS

DINNER IDEAS

STAYING *On Track*

MY WEIGHT LOSS DIARY:

WATER TRACKER

LOW CARB SNACKS

NOTES & REMINDERS

DOODLE MY MOOD

BREAKFAST IDEAS

LUNCH IDEAS

DINNER IDEAS

MEAL *Planner*

GROCERY LIST

- ☐
- ☐
- ☐
- ☐
- ☐
- ☐
- ☐
- ☐
- ☐
- ☐
- ☐
- ☐
- ☐
- ☐
- ☐
- ☐

MON

TUES

WED

THUR

FRI

SAT

SUN

KETO *Recipe*

RECIPE NAME:

	Keto	Low Carb	Paleo	Vegetarian	Vegan	Dairy Free	Gluten Free
	☐	☐	☐	☐	☐	☐	☐

QTY	INGREDIENTS	RECIPE INSTRUCTIONS

NOTES & RECIPE REVIEW

Serves	
Prep Time	
Cook Time	
Tools	
Temp	

Total	Carbs	Fat	Protein	Cals

DAILY FOOD *Tracker*

FOOD TRACKER

MEAL/SNACK	NET CARBS	FAT	CAL	PROTEIN
DAILY GOAL:				
TOTAL:				

NOTES & MEAL IDEAS

FITNESS TRACKER

		Notes
Type		
Time		
Avg HR		
Max HR		
Reps		
Cals		

DAILY OVERVIEW

		Notes		On Track
Sleep				
Water Intake				
Steps Taken				
Active Mins				Goal Met
Active Hours				
Cals Burned				

DAILY FOOD *Tracker*

FOOD TRACKER

MEAL/SNACK	NET CARBS	FAT	CAL	PROTEIN
DAILY GOAL:				
TOTAL:				

NOTES & MEAL IDEAS

FITNESS TRACKER

		Notes
Type		
Time		
Avg HR		
Max HR		
Reps		
Cals		

DAILY OVERVIEW

		Notes		
Sleep			On Track	
Water Intake				
Steps Taken				
Active Mins			Goal Met	
Active Hours				
Cals Burned				

DAILY FOOD *Tracker*

FOOD TRACKER

MEAL/SNACK	NET CARBS	FAT	CAL	PROTEIN
DAILY GOAL:				
TOTAL:				

NOTES & MEAL IDEAS

FITNESS TRACKER

		Notes
Type		
Time		
Avg HR		
Max HR		
Reps		
Cals		

DAILY OVERVIEW

		Notes		
Sleep			On Track	
Water Intake				
Steps Taken				
Active Mins			Goal Met	
Active Hours				
Cals Burned				

DAILY FOOD *Tracker*

FOOD TRACKER

MEAL/SNACK	NET CARBS	FAT	CAL	PROTEIN

DAILY GOAL:

TOTAL:

FITNESS TRACKER

		Notes
Type		
Time		
Avg HR		
Max HR		
Reps		
Cals		

DAILY OVERVIEW

		Notes		On Track
Sleep				
Water Intake				
Steps Taken				
Active Mins				Goal Met
Active Hours				
Cals Burned				

DAILY FOOD *Tracker*

FOOD TRACKER

MEAL/SNACK	NET CARBS	FAT	CAL	PROTEIN
DAILY GOAL:				
TOTAL:				

NOTES & MEAL IDEAS

FITNESS TRACKER

		Notes
Type		
Time		
Avg HR		
Max HR		
Reps		
Cals		

DAILY OVERVIEW

		Notes		
Sleep			On Track	
Water Intake				
Steps Taken				
Active Mins			Goal Met	
Active Hours				
Cals Burned				

DAILY FOOD *Tracker*

FOOD TRACKER

MEAL/SNACK	NET CARBS	FAT	CAL	PROTEIN

DAILY GOAL:

TOTAL:

NOTES & MEAL IDEAS

FITNESS TRACKER

Type		Notes
Time		
Avg HR		
Max HR		
Reps		
Cals		

DAILY OVERVIEW

Sleep		Notes		On Track
Water Intake				
Steps Taken				
Active Mins				Goal Met
Active Hours				
Cals Burned				

DAILY FOOD *Tracker*

FOOD TRACKER

MEAL/SNACK	NET CARBS	FAT	CAL	PROTEIN
DAILY GOAL:				
TOTAL:				

NOTES & MEAL IDEAS

FITNESS TRACKER

		Notes
Type		
Time		
Avg HR		
Max HR		
Reps		
Cals		

DAILY OVERVIEW

		Notes		
Sleep			On Track	
Water Intake				
Steps Taken				
Active Mins			Goal Met	
Active Hours				
Cals Burned				

KETO GO TO *Meals*

FAVORITE KETO FRIENDLY MEALS

BREAKFAST	LUNCH	DINNER	SNACKS

BREAKFAST	LUNCH	DINNER	SNACKS

BREAKFAST	LUNCH	DINNER	SNACKS

BREAKFAST	LUNCH	DINNER	SNACKS

BREAKFAST	LUNCH	DINNER	SNACKS

BREAKFAST	LUNCH	DINNER	SNACKS

BREAKFAST	LUNCH	DINNER	SNACKS

12 WEEK *Keto Meal Tracker*

12 Week Keto Challenge

MONTH	JAN	FEB	MAR	APR	MAY	JUN	JUL	AUG	SEP	OCT	NOV	DEC
WEEK	01	02	03	04	05	06	07	08	09	10	11	12

	BREAKFAST	LUNCH	DINNER	SNACKS
M				
T				
W				
T				
F				
S				
S				

GROCERY SHOPPING LIST / RECIPE INGREDIENTS

Weekly Meal Planner

Week of:

	Breakfast	Lunch	Dinner	Snack	Other
Monday	TOTAL Carbs Fat Protein Cals	TOTAL Carbs Fat Protein Cals	TOTAL Carbs Fat Protein Cals	TOTAL Carbs Fat Protein Cals	TOTAL Carbs Fat Protein Cals
Tuesday	TOTAL Carbs Fat Protein Cals	TOTAL Carbs Fat Protein Cals	TOTAL Carbs Fat Protein Cals	TOTAL Carbs Fat Protein Cals	TOTAL Carbs Fat Protein Cals
Wednesday	TOTAL Carbs Fat Protein Cals	TOTAL Carbs Fat Protein Cals	TOTAL Carbs Fat Protein Cals	TOTAL Carbs Fat Protein Cals	TOTAL Carbs Fat Protein Cals
Thursday	TOTAL Carbs Fat Protein Cals	TOTAL Carbs Fat Protein Cals	TOTAL Carbs Fat Protein Cals	TOTAL Carbs Fat Protein Cals	TOTAL Carbs Fat Protein Cals
Friday	TOTAL Carbs Fat Protein Cals	TOTAL Carbs Fat Protein Cals	TOTAL Carbs Fat Protein Cals	TOTAL Carbs Fat Protein Cals	TOTAL Carbs Fat Protein Cals
Saturday	TOTAL Carbs Fat Protein Cals	TOTAL Carbs Fat Protein Cals	TOTAL Carbs Fat Protein Cals	TOTAL Carbs Fat Protein Cals	TOTAL Carbs Fat Protein Cals
Sunday	TOTAL Carbs Fat Protein Cals	TOTAL Carbs Fat Protein Cals	TOTAL Carbs Fat Protein Cals	TOTAL Carbs Fat Protein Cals	TOTAL Carbs Fat Protein Cals

100 Days of Keto

STARTING WEIGHT:

DAY 100 WEIGHT:

1	2	3	4	5	6	7	8	9	10	**LBS LOST:** **INCHES LOST:**
11	12	13	14	15	16	17	18	19	20	**LBS LOST:** **INCHES LOST:**
21	22	23	24	25	26	27	28	29	30	**LBS LOST:** **INCHES LOST:**
31	32	33	34	35	36	37	38	39	40	**LBS LOST:** **INCHES LOST:**
41	42	43	44	45	46	47	48	49	50	**LBS LOST:** **INCHES LOST:**
51	52	53	54	55	56	57	58	59	60	**LBS LOST:** **INCHES LOST:**
61	62	63	64	65	66	67	68	69	70	**LBS LOST:** **INCHES LOST:**
71	72	73	74	75	76	77	78	79	80	**LBS LOST:** **INCHES LOST:**
81	82	83	84	85	86	87	88	89	90	**LBS LOST:** **INCHES LOST:**
91	92	93	94	95	96	97	98	99	100	**LBS LOST:** **INCHES LOST:**

TOTAL WEIGHT LOST:

TOTAL INCHES LOST:

NOTES & REFLECTIONS:

24 DAY *Weight Loss Steps*

WEIGHT LOSS PLAN OF ACTION:

PERSONAL ACCOMPLISHMENTS

30 DAY *Keto Challenge*

- [ ]
- [ ]
- [ ]
- [ ]
- [ ]
- [ ]
- [ ]
- [ ]
- [ ]
- [ ]
- [ ]
- [ ]
- [ ]
- [ ]
- [ ]
- [ ]
- [ ]

INSPIRATIONAL REMINDERS

STARTED >

FINISHED >

1	2	3	4	5	6	7	8	9	10
11	12	13	14	15	16	17	18	19	20
21	22	23	24	25	26	27	28	29	30

30-DAY KETO RESULTS

PERSONAL ACCOMPLISHMENTS

60 Days of Keto

STARTING WEIGHT: **DAY 60 WEIGHT:**

| 1 | 2 | 3 | 4 | 5 | 6 | 7 | 8 | 9 | 10 |

LBS LOST:
INCHES LOST:

| 11 | 12 | 13 | 14 | 15 | 16 | 17 | 18 | 19 | 20 |

LBS LOST:
INCHES LOST:

| 21 | 22 | 23 | 24 | 25 | 26 | 27 | 28 | 29 | 30 |

LBS LOST:
INCHES LOST:

| 31 | 32 | 33 | 34 | 35 | 36 | 37 | 38 | 39 | 40 |

LBS LOST:
INCHES LOST:

| 41 | 42 | 43 | 44 | 45 | 46 | 47 | 48 | 49 | 50 |

LBS LOST:
INCHES LOST:

| 51 | 52 | 53 | 54 | 55 | 56 | 57 | 58 | 59 | 60 |

LBS LOST:
INCHES LOST:

TOTAL WEIGHT LOST: **TOTAL INCHES LOST:**

NOTES & REFLECTIONS:

30 Days of Keto

STARTING WEIGHT:

DAY 30 WEIGHT:

| 1 | 2 | 3 | 4 | 5 | 6 | 7 | 8 | 9 | 10 |

LBS LOST:

INCHES LOST:

| 11 | 12 | 13 | 14 | 15 | 16 | 17 | 18 | 19 | 20 |

LBS LOST:

INCHES LOST:

| 21 | 22 | 23 | 24 | 25 | 26 | 27 | 28 | 29 | 30 |

LBS LOST:

INCHES LOST:

TOTAL WEIGHT LOST:

TOTAL INCHES LOST:

NOTES:

PERSONAL ACCOMPLISHMENTS:

THOUGHTS & REFLECTIONS:

WEIGHT LOSS *Journal*

MONDAY

TUESDAY

WEDNESDAY

THURSDAY

FRIDAY

SATURDAY

SUNDAY

WEEK OF:

DATE	WEIGHT LOSS ACTION PLAN

NOTES

WEEKLY *Fasting Tracker*

Week Of: _____

MONDAY

Goal	12	1	2	3	4	5	6	7	8	9	10	11	12	1	2	3	4	5	6	7	8	9	10	11
Actual	12	1	2	3	4	5	6	7	8	9	10	11	12	1	2	3	4	5	6	7	8	9	10	11

TUESDAY

Goal	12	1	2	3	4	5	6	7	8	9	10	11	12	1	2	3	4	5	6	7	8	9	10	11
Actual	12	1	2	3	4	5	6	7	8	9	10	11	12	1	2	3	4	5	6	7	8	9	10	11

WEDNESDAY

Goal	12	1	2	3	4	5	6	7	8	9	10	11	12	1	2	3	4	5	6	7	8	9	10	11
Actual	12	1	2	3	4	5	6	7	8	9	10	11	12	1	2	3	4	5	6	7	8	9	10	11

THURSDAY

Goal	12	1	2	3	4	5	6	7	8	9	10	11	12	1	2	3	4	5	6	7	8	9	10	11
Actual	12	1	2	3	4	5	6	7	8	9	10	11	12	1	2	3	4	5	6	7	8	9	10	11

FRIDAY

Goal	12	1	2	3	4	5	6	7	8	9	10	11	12	1	2	3	4	5	6	7	8	9	10	11
Actual	12	1	2	3	4	5	6	7	8	9	10	11	12	1	2	3	4	5	6	7	8	9	10	11

SATURDAY

Goal	12	1	2	3	4	5	6	7	8	9	10	11	12	1	2	3	4	5	6	7	8	9	10	11
Actual	12	1	2	3	4	5	6	7	8	9	10	11	12	1	2	3	4	5	6	7	8	9	10	11

SUNDAY

Goal	12	1	2	3	4	5	6	7	8	9	10	11	12	1	2	3	4	5	6	7	8	9	10	11
Actual	12	1	2	3	4	5	6	7	8	9	10	11	12	1	2	3	4	5	6	7	8	9	10	11

21 DAY KETO *Challenge*

It takes just 21 days to create a healthy routine that will last a lifetime!

START DATE	END DATE

1	2	3	4	5
6	7	8	9	10
11	12	13	14	15
16	17	18	19	20

21	NOTES

Keto Grocery Inventory

DATE: _____

QTY	PRODUCE

QTY	MEAT & FISH

QTY	FROZEN FOODS

QTY	DAIRY

QTY	PANTRY

QTY	OTHER/MISC.

WEIGHT LOSS *Journal*

MONDAY

TUESDAY

WEDNESDAY

THURSDAY

FRIDAY

SATURDAY

SUNDAY

WEEK OF:

DATE	WEIGHT LOSS ACTION PLAN

NOTES

WEIGHT LOSS *Tracker*

MONTHLY GOAL

_____

DATE: _____ _____ _____ _____ _____

BUST					
WAIST					
HIPS					
BICEP					
THIGH					
CALF					
WEIGHT					

TOTAL WEIGHT LOSS >>

MONTHLY PROGRESS *Tracker*

JAN   FEB   MAR   APR   MAY   JUN   JUL   AUG   SEP   OCT   NOV   DEC

MON	TUE	WED	THU	FRI	SAT	SUN

WEIGHT LOSS MILESTONE TRACKER

CHEAT DAY TRACKER

WEEKLY DIET SUCCESS TRACKER & NOTES

MY WEIGHT LOSS *Routine*

CREATING A ROUTINE FOR SUCCESS

WEIGHT LOSS SUCCESS: HABIT & ROUTINE TRACKER	
DRINK LOTS OF WATER TODAY	**TRACK TOTAL CARB INTAKE**

COMPLETE TOP 3 GOALS OF THE DAY

1
2
3

PLAN MY MEALS FOR THE DAY:

BREAKFAST	LUNCH	DINNER

DAILY TRACKER & TO DO LIST	ACCOMPLISHMENTS

NOTES

MY KETO *Routine*

Morning   *My Weight Loss Routine*   m t w t f s s

Mid Day   *My Weight Loss Routine*   m t w t f s s

Evening   *My Weight Loss Routine*   m t w t f s s

Night   *My Weight Loss Routine*   m t w t f s s

WEEKLY *Fasting Tracker*

Week Of: _____

MONDAY

Goal	12	1	2	3	4	5	6	7	8	9	10	11	12	1	2	3	4	5	6	7	8	9	10	11
Actual	12	1	2	3	4	5	6	7	8	9	10	11	12	1	2	3	4	5	6	7	8	9	10	11

TUESDAY

Goal	12	1	2	3	4	5	6	7	8	9	10	11	12	1	2	3	4	5	6	7	8	9	10	11
Actual	12	1	2	3	4	5	6	7	8	9	10	11	12	1	2	3	4	5	6	7	8	9	10	11

WEDNESDAY

Goal	12	1	2	3	4	5	6	7	8	9	10	11	12	1	2	3	4	5	6	7	8	9	10	11
Actual	12	1	2	3	4	5	6	7	8	9	10	11	12	1	2	3	4	5	6	7	8	9	10	11

THURSDAY

Goal	12	1	2	3	4	5	6	7	8	9	10	11	12	1	2	3	4	5	6	7	8	9	10	11
Actual	12	1	2	3	4	5	6	7	8	9	10	11	12	1	2	3	4	5	6	7	8	9	10	11

FRIDAY

Goal	12	1	2	3	4	5	6	7	8	9	10	11	12	1	2	3	4	5	6	7	8	9	10	11
Actual	12	1	2	3	4	5	6	7	8	9	10	11	12	1	2	3	4	5	6	7	8	9	10	11

SATURDAY

Goal	12	1	2	3	4	5	6	7	8	9	10	11	12	1	2	3	4	5	6	7	8	9	10	11
Actual	12	1	2	3	4	5	6	7	8	9	10	11	12	1	2	3	4	5	6	7	8	9	10	11

SUNDAY

Goal	12	1	2	3	4	5	6	7	8	9	10	11	12	1	2	3	4	5	6	7	8	9	10	11
Actual	12	1	2	3	4	5	6	7	8	9	10	11	12	1	2	3	4	5	6	7	8	9	10	11

KETO *Meal* LOG BOOK

	BREAKFAST	LUNCH	DINNER	SNACKS
MONDAY				
TUESDAY				
WEDNESDAY				
THURSDAY				
FRIDAY				
SATURDAY				
SUNDAY				

MY PROGRESS *Tracker*

SLEEP TRACKER:

DATE _____

RISE:		BEDTIME:		SLEEP (HRS):

NOTES FOR THE DAY

_____

_____

_____

IN A STATE OF KETOSIS?

YES   NO   UNSURE

WATER INTAKE TRACKER

EXERCISE / WORKOUT ROUTINE

DAILY ENERGY LEVEL

HIGH	**MEDIUM**	**LOW**

BREAKFAST

FAT: CARBS: PROTEIN: CALORIES:

LUNCH

FAT: CARBS: PROTEIN: CALORIES:

DINNER

FAT: CARBS: PROTEIN: CALORIES:

SNACKS

FAT: CARBS: PROTEIN: CALORIES:

TOP 6 PRIORITIES OF THE DAY

END OF THE DAY TOTAL OVERVIEW

CARBS	FAT	PROTEIN	CALORIES

Macro Quick Reference

MACRO TRACKER

QTY	TYPE	PROTEIN	FAT	CARBS	CALS	NOTES

INTERMITTENT *Fasting Log*

WEEK OF:

	START TIME	END TIME	TOTAL FAST HRS
M	:	:	:
T	:	:	:
W	:	:	:
T	:	:	:
F	:	:	:
S	:	:	:
S	:	:	:

WEEK OF:

	START TIME	END TIME	TOTAL FAST HRS
M	:	:	:
T	:	:	:
W	:	:	:
T	:	:	:
F	:	:	:
S	:	:	:
S	:	:	:

WEEK OF:

	START TIME	END TIME	TOTAL FAST HRS
M	:	:	:
T	:	:	:
W	:	:	:
T	:	:	:
F	:	:	:
S	:	:	:
S	:	:	:

WEEK OF:

	START TIME	END TIME	TOTAL FAST HRS
M	:	:	:
T	:	:	:
W	:	:	:
T	:	:	:
F	:	:	:
S	:	:	:
S	:	:	:

WEEK OF:

	START TIME	END TIME	TOTAL FAST HRS
M	:	:	:
T	:	:	:
W	:	:	:
T	:	:	:
F	:	:	:
S	:	:	:
S	:	:	:

WEEK OF:

	START TIME	END TIME	TOTAL FAST HRS
M	:	:	:
T	:	:	:
W	:	:	:
T	:	:	:
F	:	:	:
S	:	:	:
S	:	:	:

MILESTONES & ACCOMPLISHMENTS

NOTES & REFLECTIONS

GOALS & *Accomplishments*

Month | JAN FEB MAR APR MAY JUN JUL AUG SEP OCT NOV DEC

THIS MONTH'S **GOALS**

ACTION PLAN

M T W T F S S

NOTES:

WEEKLY GOALS

M

T

W

T

F

S

S

THOUGHTS

MEALS:	BREAKFAST	LUNCH	DINNER	SNACKS
M				
T				
W				
T				
F				
S				
S				

Low Carb Shopping List

FRESH PRODUCE

MEAT AND SEAFOOD

DAIRY PRODUCTS

PANTRY ITEMS

FROZEN / OTHER

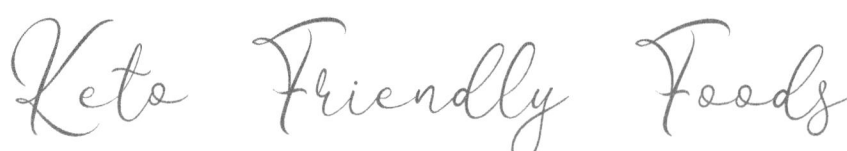

Keto Friendly Foods

KETO FRIENDLY FOODS	NET CARBS	PROTEINS	FAT

FOODS TO EAT IN MODERATION	NET CARBS	PROTEINS	FAT

STAYING *On Track*

MY WEIGHT LOSS DIARY:

_____

_____

_____

_____

WATER TRACKER

NOTES & REMINDERS

DOODLE MY MOOD

LOW CARB SNACKS

BREAKFAST IDEAS

LUNCH IDEAS

DINNER IDEAS

STAYING *On Track*

MY WEIGHT LOSS DIARY:

WATER TRACKER

LOW CARB SNACKS

NOTES & REMINDERS

DOODLE MY MOOD

BREAKFAST IDEAS

LUNCH IDEAS

DINNER IDEAS

STAYING *On Track*

MY WEIGHT LOSS DIARY:

_____

_____

_____

_____

WATER TRACKER

NOTES & REMINDERS

DOODLE MY MOOD

LOW CARB SNACKS

BREAKFAST IDEAS

LUNCH IDEAS

DINNER IDEAS

STAYING *On Track*

MY WEIGHT LOSS DIARY:

WATER TRACKER

ᗉ ᗉ ᗉ ᗉ ᗉ ᗉ ᗉ ᗉ

LOW CARB SNACKS

NOTES & REMINDERS

DOODLE MY MOOD

BREAKFAST IDEAS

LUNCH IDEAS

DINNER IDEAS

STAYING *On Track*

MY WEIGHT LOSS DIARY:

_____

_____

_____

_____

WATER TRACKER

NOTES & REMINDERS

DOODLE MY MOOD

LOW CARB SNACKS

BREAKFAST IDEAS

LUNCH IDEAS

DINNER IDEAS

STAYING *On Track*

MY WEIGHT LOSS DIARY:

WATER TRACKER

NOTES & REMINDERS

DOODLE MY MOOD

LOW CARB SNACKS

BREAKFAST IDEAS

LUNCH IDEAS

DINNER IDEAS

STAYING *On Track*

MY WEIGHT LOSS DIARY:

WATER TRACKER

LOW CARB SNACKS

NOTES & REMINDERS

DOODLE MY MOOD

BREAKFAST IDEAS

LUNCH IDEAS

DINNER IDEAS

MEAL *Planner*

GROCERY LIST

MON

TUES

WED

THUR

FRI

SAT

SUN

KETO *Recipe*

RECIPE NAME:

_____

	Keto	Low Carb	Paleo	Vegetarian	Vegan	Dairy Free	Gluten Free
	☐	☐	☐	☐	☐	☐	☐

QTY	INGREDIENTS	RECIPE INSTRUCTIONS

NOTES & RECIPE REVIEW

Serves	
Prep Time	
Cook Time	
Tools	
Temp	

Total	Carbs	Fat	Protein	Cals

DAILY FOOD *Tracker*

FOOD TRACKER

MEAL/SNACK	NET CARBS	FAT	CAL	PROTEIN

DAILY GOAL:

TOTAL:

NOTES & MEAL IDEAS

FITNESS TRACKER

		Notes
Type		
Time		
Avg HR		
Max HR		
Reps		
Cals		

DAILY OVERVIEW

		Notes		On Track
Sleep				
Water Intake				
Steps Taken				
Active Mins				Goal Met
Active Hours				
Cals Burned				

DAILY FOOD *Tracker*

FOOD TRACKER

MEAL/SNACK	NET CARBS	FAT	CAL	PROTEIN
DAILY GOAL:				
TOTAL:				

NOTES & MEAL IDEAS

FITNESS TRACKER

		Notes
Type		
Time		
Avg HR		
Max HR		
Reps		
Cals		

DAILY OVERVIEW

		Notes		On Track
Sleep				
Water Intake				
Steps Taken				
Active Mins				Goal Met
Active Hours				
Cals Burned				

DAILY FOOD *Tracker*

FOOD TRACKER

MEAL/SNACK	NET CARBS	FAT	CAL	PROTEIN
DAILY GOAL:				
TOTAL:				

NOTES & MEAL IDEAS

FITNESS TRACKER

Type		Notes
Time		
Avg HR		
Max HR		
Reps		
Cals		

DAILY OVERVIEW

Sleep		Notes
Water Intake		
Steps Taken		
Active Mins		
Active Hours		
Cals Burned		

On Track

Goal Met

DAILY FOOD *Tracker*

FOOD TRACKER

MEAL/SNACK	NET CARBS	FAT	CAL	PROTEIN
DAILY GOAL:				
TOTAL:				

NOTES & MEAL IDEAS

FITNESS TRACKER

Type		Notes
Time		
Avg HR		
Max HR		
Reps		
Cals		

DAILY OVERVIEW

Sleep		Notes		On Track
Water Intake				
Steps Taken				
Active Mins				Goal Met
Active Hours				
Cals Burned				

DAILY FOOD *Tracker*

FOOD TRACKER

MEAL/SNACK	NET CARBS	FAT	CAL	PROTEIN
DAILY GOAL:				
TOTAL:				

NOTES & MEAL IDEAS

FITNESS TRACKER

Type		Notes
Time		
Avg HR		
Max HR		
Reps		
Cals		

DAILY OVERVIEW

Sleep		Notes		On Track
Water Intake				
Steps Taken				
Active Mins				Goal Met
Active Hours				
Cals Burned				

DAILY FOOD *Tracker*

FOOD TRACKER

MEAL/SNACK	NET CARBS	FAT	CAL	PROTEIN
DAILY GOAL:				
TOTAL:				

NOTES & MEAL IDEAS

FITNESS TRACKER

Type		Notes
Time		
Avg HR		
Max HR		
Reps		
Cals		

DAILY OVERVIEW

Sleep		Notes		On Track
Water Intake				
Steps Taken				
Active Mins				
Active Hours				Goal Met
Cals Burned				

DAILY FOOD *Tracker*

FOOD TRACKER

MEAL/SNACK	NET CARBS	FAT	CAL	PROTEIN

DAILY GOAL:

TOTAL:

NOTES & MEAL IDEAS

FITNESS TRACKER

Type	
Time	
Avg HR	
Max HR	
Reps	
Cals	

Notes

DAILY OVERVIEW

Sleep	
Water Intake	
Steps Taken	
Active Mins	
Active Hours	
Cals Burned	

Notes

On Track

Goal Met

KETO GO TO *Meals*

BREAKFAST	LUNCH	DINNER	SNACKS
BREAKFAST	LUNCH	DINNER	SNACKS
BREAKFAST	LUNCH	DINNER	SNACKS
BREAKFAST	LUNCH	DINNER	SNACKS
BREAKFAST	LUNCH	DINNER	SNACKS
BREAKFAST	LUNCH	DINNER	SNACKS
BREAKFAST	LUNCH	DINNER	SNACKS

12 WEEK *Keto Meal Tracker*

MONTH	JAN	FEB	MAR	APR	MAY	JUN	JUL	AUG	SEP	OCT	NOV	DEC
WEEK	01	02	03	04	05	06	07	08	09	10	11	12

	BREAKFAST	LUNCH	DINNER	SNACKS
M				
T				
W				
T				
F				
S				
S				

GROCERY SHOPPING LIST / RECIPE INGREDIENTS

Weekly Meal Planner

Week of: _____

	Breakfast	Lunch	Dinner	Snack	Other
Monday	TOTAL Carbs Fat Protein Cals	TOTAL Carbs Fat Protein Cals	TOTAL Carbs Fat Protein Cals	TOTAL Carbs Fat Protein Cals	TOTAL Carbs Fat Protein Cals
Tuesday	TOTAL Carbs Fat Protein Cals	TOTAL Carbs Fat Protein Cals	TOTAL Carbs Fat Protein Cals	TOTAL Carbs Fat Protein Cals	TOTAL Carbs Fat Protein Cals
Wednesday	TOTAL Carbs Fat Protein Cals	TOTAL Carbs Fat Protein Cals	TOTAL Carbs Fat Protein Cals	TOTAL Carbs Fat Protein Cals	TOTAL Carbs Fat Protein Cals
Thursday	TOTAL Carbs Fat Protein Cals	TOTAL Carbs Fat Protein Cals	TOTAL Carbs Fat Protein Cals	TOTAL Carbs Fat Protein Cals	TOTAL Carbs Fat Protein Cals
Friday	TOTAL Carbs Fat Protein Cals	TOTAL Carbs Fat Protein Cals	TOTAL Carbs Fat Protein Cals	TOTAL Carbs Fat Protein Cals	TOTAL Carbs Fat Protein Cals
Saturday	TOTAL Carbs Fat Protein Cals	TOTAL Carbs Fat Protein Cals	TOTAL Carbs Fat Protein Cals	TOTAL Carbs Fat Protein Cals	TOTAL Carbs Fat Protein Cals
Sunday	TOTAL Carbs Fat Protein Cals	TOTAL Carbs Fat Protein Cals	TOTAL Carbs Fat Protein Cals	TOTAL Carbs Fat Protein Cals	TOTAL Carbs Fat Protein Cals

WEIGHT LOSS *Journal*

MONDAY

TUESDAY

WEDNESDAY

THURSDAY

FRIDAY

SATURDAY

SUNDAY

WEEK OF:

DATE	WEIGHT LOSS ACTION PLAN

NOTES

MY WEIGHT LOSS *Routine*

CREATING A ROUTINE FOR SUCCESS

WEIGHT LOSS SUCCESS: HABIT & ROUTINE TRACKER	
DRINK LOTS OF WATER TODAY	TRACK TOTAL CARB INTAKE

COMPLETE TOP 3 GOALS OF THE DAY

1

2

3

PLAN MY MEALS FOR THE DAY:

BREAKFAST	LUNCH	DINNER

DAILY TRACKER & TO DO LIST	ACCOMPLISHMENTS

NOTES

MY KETO *Routine*

Morning	My Weight Loss Routine	m t w t f s s

Mid Day	My Weight Loss Routine	m t w t f s s

Evening	My Weight Loss Routine	m t w t f s s

Night	My Weight Loss Routine	m t w t f s s

WEEKLY *Fasting Tracker*

Week Of: _____

MONDAY

Goal	12	1	2	3	4	5	6	7	8	9	10	11	12	1	2	3	4	5	6	7	8	9	10	11
Actual	12	1	2	3	4	5	6	7	8	9	10	11	12	1	2	3	4	5	6	7	8	9	10	11

TUESDAY

Goal	12	1	2	3	4	5	6	7	8	9	10	11	12	1	2	3	4	5	6	7	8	9	10	11
Actual	12	1	2	3	4	5	6	7	8	9	10	11	12	1	2	3	4	5	6	7	8	9	10	11

WEDNESDAY

Goal	12	1	2	3	4	5	6	7	8	9	10	11	12	1	2	3	4	5	6	7	8	9	10	11
Actual	12	1	2	3	4	5	6	7	8	9	10	11	12	1	2	3	4	5	6	7	8	9	10	11

THURSDAY

Goal	12	1	2	3	4	5	6	7	8	9	10	11	12	1	2	3	4	5	6	7	8	9	10	11
Actual	12	1	2	3	4	5	6	7	8	9	10	11	12	1	2	3	4	5	6	7	8	9	10	11

FRIDAY

Goal	12	1	2	3	4	5	6	7	8	9	10	11	12	1	2	3	4	5	6	7	8	9	10	11
Actual	12	1	2	3	4	5	6	7	8	9	10	11	12	1	2	3	4	5	6	7	8	9	10	11

SATURDAY

Goal	12	1	2	3	4	5	6	7	8	9	10	11	12	1	2	3	4	5	6	7	8	9	10	11
Actual	12	1	2	3	4	5	6	7	8	9	10	11	12	1	2	3	4	5	6	7	8	9	10	11

SUNDAY

Goal	12	1	2	3	4	5	6	7	8	9	10	11	12	1	2	3	4	5	6	7	8	9	10	11
Actual	12	1	2	3	4	5	6	7	8	9	10	11	12	1	2	3	4	5	6	7	8	9	10	11

KETO *Meal* LOG BOOK

	BREAKFAST	LUNCH	DINNER	SNACKS
MONDAY				
TUESDAY				
WEDNESDAY				
THURSDAY				
FRIDAY				
SATURDAY				
SUNDAY				

MY PROGRESS *Tracker*

SLEEP TRACKER:

DATE ....

☀ RISE: [ ] 🌙 BEDTIME: [ ] 💭 SLEEP (HRS): [ ]

NOTES FOR THE DAY

....

....

....

EXERCISE / WORKOUT ROUTINE

[ ]

TOP 6 PRIORITIES OF THE DAY

....

....

....

IN A STATE OF KETOSIS?

YES   NO   UNSURE

WATER INTAKE TRACKER

DAILY ENERGY LEVEL

HIGH	**MEDIUM**	**LOW**

BREAKFAST

FAT: CARBS: PROTEIN: CALORIES:

LUNCH

FAT: CARBS: PROTEIN: CALORIES:

DINNER

FAT: CARBS: PROTEIN: CALORIES:

SNACKS

FAT: CARBS: PROTEIN: CALORIES:

END OF THE DAY TOTAL OVERVIEW

CARBS	FAT	PROTEIN	CALORIES
[ ]	[ ]	[ ]	[ ]

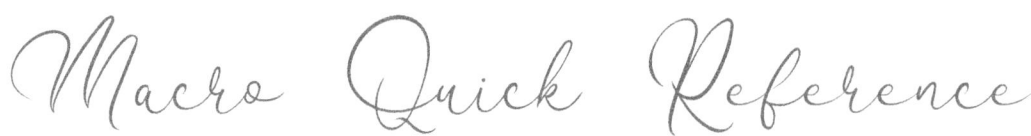

Macro Quick Reference

MACRO TRACKER

QTY	TYPE	PROTEIN	FAT	CARBS	CALS	NOTES

INTERMITTENT *Fasting Log*

WEEK OF:

	START TIME	END TIME	TOTAL FAST HRS
M	:	:	:
T	:	:	:
W	:	:	:
T	:	:	:
F	:	:	:
S	:	:	:
S	:	:	:

WEEK OF:

	START TIME	END TIME	TOTAL FAST HRS
M	:	:	:
T	:	:	:
W	:	:	:
T	:	:	:
F	:	:	:
S	:	:	:
S	:	:	:

WEEK OF:

	START TIME	END TIME	TOTAL FAST HRS
M	:	:	:
T	:	:	:
W	:	:	:
T	:	:	:
F	:	:	:
S	:	:	:
S	:	:	:

WEEK OF:

	START TIME	END TIME	TOTAL FAST HRS
M	:	:	:
T	:	:	:
W	:	:	:
T	:	:	:
F	:	:	:
S	:	:	:
S	:	:	:

WEEK OF:

	START TIME	END TIME	TOTAL FAST HRS
M	:	:	:
T	:	:	:
W	:	:	:
T	:	:	:
F	:	:	:
S	:	:	:
S	:	:	:

WEEK OF:

	START TIME	END TIME	TOTAL FAST HRS
M	:	:	:
T	:	:	:
W	:	:	:
T	:	:	:
F	:	:	:
S	:	:	:
S	:	:	:

MILESTONES & ACCOMPLISHMENTS

NOTES & REFLECTIONS

GOALS & *Accomplishments*

THIS MONTH'S **GOALS**

ACTION PLAN

M T W T F S S

WEEKLY GOALS

M

T

W

T

F

S

S

NOTES:

THOUGHTS

MEALS:	BREAKFAST	LUNCH	DINNER	SNACKS
M				
T				
W				
T				
F				
S				
S				

Low Carb Shopping List

FRESH PRODUCE

MEAT AND SEAFOOD

DAIRY PRODUCTS

PANTRY ITEMS

FROZEN / OTHER

Keto Friendly Foods

KETO FRIENDLY FOODS	NET CARBS	PROTEINS	FAT

FOODS TO EAT IN MODERATION	NET CARBS	PROTEINS	FAT

STAYING *On Track*

MY WEIGHT LOSS DIARY:

_____

_____

_____

_____

WATER TRACKER

NOTES & REMINDERS

DOODLE MY MOOD

LOW CARB SNACKS

BREAKFAST IDEAS

LUNCH IDEAS

DINNER IDEAS

STAYING *On Track*

MY WEIGHT LOSS DIARY:

WATER TRACKER

LOW CARB SNACKS

NOTES & REMINDERS

DOODLE MY MOOD

BREAKFAST IDEAS

LUNCH IDEAS

DINNER IDEAS

STAYING *On Track*

MY WEIGHT LOSS DIARY:

_____

_____

_____

_____

WATER TRACKER

○ ○ ○ ○ ○ ○ ○

LOW CARB SNACKS

NOTES & REMINDERS

DOODLE MY MOOD

BREAKFAST IDEAS

LUNCH IDEAS

DINNER IDEAS

STAYING *On Track*

MY WEIGHT LOSS DIARY:

WATER TRACKER

LOW CARB SNACKS

NOTES & REMINDERS

DOODLE MY MOOD

BREAKFAST IDEAS

LUNCH IDEAS

DINNER IDEAS

STAYING *On Track*

MY WEIGHT LOSS DIARY:

_____

_____

_____

_____

WATER TRACKER

NOTES & REMINDERS

DOODLE MY MOOD

LOW CARB SNACKS

BREAKFAST IDEAS

LUNCH IDEAS

DINNER IDEAS

STAYING *On Track*

MY WEIGHT LOSS DIARY:

WATER TRACKER

LOW CARB SNACKS

NOTES & REMINDERS

DOODLE MY MOOD

BREAKFAST IDEAS

LUNCH IDEAS

DINNER IDEAS

STAYING *On Track*

MY WEIGHT LOSS DIARY:

_____

_____

_____

_____

WATER TRACKER

⬡ ⬡ ⬡ ⬡ ⬡ ⬡ ⬡

LOW CARB SNACKS

NOTES & REMINDERS

DOODLE MY MOOD

BREAKFAST IDEAS

LUNCH IDEAS

DINNER IDEAS

MEAL *Planner*

GROCERY LIST

WEEK OF

MON

TUES

WED

THUR

FRI

SAT

SUN

KETO *Recipe*

RECIPE NAME:

Keto	Low Carb	Paleo	Vegetarian	Vegan	Dairy Free	Gluten Free
☐	☐	☐	☐	☐	☐	☐

QTY	INGREDIENTS

RECIPE INSTRUCTIONS

NOTES & RECIPE REVIEW

Serves	
Prep Time	
Cook Time	
Tools	
Temp	

Total	Carbs	Fat	Protein	Cals

DAILY FOOD *Tracker*

FOOD TRACKER

MEAL/SNACK	NET CARBS	FAT	CAL	PROTEIN
DAILY GOAL:				
TOTAL:				

NOTES & MEAL IDEAS

FITNESS TRACKER

Type		Notes
Time		
Avg HR		
Max HR		
Reps		
Cals		

DAILY OVERVIEW

Sleep		Notes		On Track
Water Intake				
Steps Taken				
Active Mins				Goal Met
Active Hours				
Cals Burned				

DAILY FOOD *Tracker*

FOOD TRACKER

MEAL/SNACK	NET CARBS	FAT	CAL	PROTEIN
DAILY GOAL:				
TOTAL:				

NOTES & MEAL IDEAS

FITNESS TRACKER

		Notes
Type		
Time		
Avg HR		
Max HR		
Reps		
Cals		

DAILY OVERVIEW

		Notes		
Sleep			On Track	
Water Intake				
Steps Taken				
Active Mins			Goal Met	
Active Hours				
Cals Burned				

DAILY FOOD *Tracker*

FOOD TRACKER

MEAL/SNACK	NET CARBS	FAT	CAL	PROTEIN

DAILY GOAL:

TOTAL:

NOTES & MEAL IDEAS

FITNESS TRACKER

Type		Notes
Time		
Avg HR		
Max HR		
Reps		
Cals		

DAILY OVERVIEW

Sleep		Notes		On Track
Water Intake				
Steps Taken				
Active Mins				Goal Met
Active Hours				
Cals Burned				

DAILY FOOD *Tracker*

FOOD TRACKER

MEAL/SNACK	NET CARBS	FAT	CAL	PROTEIN
DAILY GOAL:				
TOTAL:				

NOTES & MEAL IDEAS

FITNESS TRACKER

		Notes
Type		
Time		
Avg HR		
Max HR		
Reps		
Cals		

DAILY OVERVIEW

		Notes		
Sleep			On Track	
Water Intake				
Steps Taken				
Active Mins			Goal Met	
Active Hours				
Cals Burned				

DAILY FOOD *Tracker*

FOOD TRACKER

MEAL/SNACK	NET CARBS	FAT	CAL	PROTEIN
DAILY GOAL:				
TOTAL:				

NOTES & MEAL IDEAS

FITNESS TRACKER

Type		Notes
Time		
Avg HR		
Max HR		
Reps		
Cals		

DAILY OVERVIEW

Sleep		Notes		On Track
Water Intake				
Steps Taken				
Active Mins				Goal Met
Active Hours				
Cals Burned				

DAILY FOOD *Tracker*

FOOD TRACKER

MEAL/SNACK	NET CARBS	FAT	CAL	PROTEIN
DAILY GOAL:				
TOTAL:				

NOTES & MEAL IDEAS

FITNESS TRACKER

Type		Notes
Time		
Avg HR		
Max HR		
Reps		
Cals		

DAILY OVERVIEW

Sleep		Notes		On Track
Water Intake				
Steps Taken				
Active Mins				Goal Met
Active Hours				
Cals Burned				

DAILY FOOD *Tracker*

FOOD TRACKER

MEAL/SNACK	NET CARBS	FAT	CAL	PROTEIN

DAILY GOAL:

TOTAL:

NOTES & MEAL IDEAS

FITNESS TRACKER

Type		Notes
Time		
Avg HR		
Max HR		
Reps		
Cals		

DAILY OVERVIEW

Sleep		Notes	On Track
Water Intake			
Steps Taken			
Active Mins			Goal Met
Active Hours			
Cals Burned			

KETO GO TO *Meals*

BREAKFAST	LUNCH	DINNER	SNACKS

BREAKFAST	LUNCH	DINNER	SNACKS

BREAKFAST	LUNCH	DINNER	SNACKS

BREAKFAST	LUNCH	DINNER	SNACKS

BREAKFAST	LUNCH	DINNER	SNACKS

BREAKFAST	LUNCH	DINNER	SNACKS

BREAKFAST	LUNCH	DINNER	SNACKS

12 WEEK *Keto Meal Tracker*

MONTH	JAN	FEB	MAR	APR	MAY	JUN	JUL	AUG	SEP	OCT	NOV	DEC
WEEK	01	02	03	04	05	06	07	08	09	10	11	12

	BREAKFAST	LUNCH	DINNER	SNACKS
M				
T				
W				
T				
F				
S				
S				

GROCERY SHOPPING LIST / RECIPE INGREDIENTS

Weekly Meal Planner

Week of: _____

	Breakfast	Lunch	Dinner	Snack	Other
Monday	TOTAL Carbs Fat Protein Cals	TOTAL Carbs Fat Protein Cals	TOTAL Carbs Fat Protein Cals	TOTAL Carbs Fat Protein Cals	TOTAL Carbs Fat Protein Cals
Tuesday	TOTAL Carbs Fat Protein Cals	TOTAL Carbs Fat Protein Cals	TOTAL Carbs Fat Protein Cals	TOTAL Carbs Fat Protein Cals	TOTAL Carbs Fat Protein Cals
Wednesday	TOTAL Carbs Fat Protein Cals	TOTAL Carbs Fat Protein Cals	TOTAL Carbs Fat Protein Cals	TOTAL Carbs Fat Protein Cals	TOTAL Carbs Fat Protein Cals
Thursday	TOTAL Carbs Fat Protein Cals	TOTAL Carbs Fat Protein Cals	TOTAL Carbs Fat Protein Cals	TOTAL Carbs Fat Protein Cals	TOTAL Carbs Fat Protein Cals
Friday	TOTAL Carbs Fat Protein Cals	TOTAL Carbs Fat Protein Cals	TOTAL Carbs Fat Protein Cals	TOTAL Carbs Fat Protein Cals	TOTAL Carbs Fat Protein Cals
Saturday	TOTAL Carbs Fat Protein Cals	TOTAL Carbs Fat Protein Cals	TOTAL Carbs Fat Protein Cals	TOTAL Carbs Fat Protein Cals	TOTAL Carbs Fat Protein Cals
Sunday	TOTAL Carbs Fat Protein Cals	TOTAL Carbs Fat Protein Cals	TOTAL Carbs Fat Protein Cals	TOTAL Carbs Fat Protein Cals	TOTAL Carbs Fat Protein Cals

WEIGHT LOSS *Journal*

MONDAY

WEEK OF:

DATE	WEIGHT LOSS ACTION PLAN

TUESDAY

WEDNESDAY

THURSDAY

FRIDAY

NOTES

SATURDAY

SUNDAY

MY WEIGHT LOSS *Routine*

WEIGHT LOSS SUCCESS: HABIT & ROUTINE TRACKER	
DRINK LOTS OF WATER TODAY	TRACK TOTAL CARB INTAKE

COMPLETE TOP 3 GOALS OF THE DAY

1

2

3

PLAN MY MEALS FOR THE DAY:

BREAKFAST	LUNCH	DINNER

DAILY TRACKER & TO DO LIST	ACCOMPLISHMENTS

NOTES

WEEKLY *Fasting Tracker*

Week Of: _____

MONDAY

Goal	12	1	2	3	4	5	6	7	8	9	10	11	12	1	2	3	4	5	6	7	8	9	10	11
Actual	12	1	2	3	4	5	6	7	8	9	10	11	12	1	2	3	4	5	6	7	8	9	10	11

TUESDAY

Goal	12	1	2	3	4	5	6	7	8	9	10	11	12	1	2	3	4	5	6	7	8	9	10	11
Actual	12	1	2	3	4	5	6	7	8	9	10	11	12	1	2	3	4	5	6	7	8	9	10	11

WEDNESDAY

Goal	12	1	2	3	4	5	6	7	8	9	10	11	12	1	2	3	4	5	6	7	8	9	10	11
Actual	12	1	2	3	4	5	6	7	8	9	10	11	12	1	2	3	4	5	6	7	8	9	10	11

THURSDAY

Goal	12	1	2	3	4	5	6	7	8	9	10	11	12	1	2	3	4	5	6	7	8	9	10	11
Actual	12	1	2	3	4	5	6	7	8	9	10	11	12	1	2	3	4	5	6	7	8	9	10	11

FRIDAY

Goal	12	1	2	3	4	5	6	7	8	9	10	11	12	1	2	3	4	5	6	7	8	9	10	11
Actual	12	1	2	3	4	5	6	7	8	9	10	11	12	1	2	3	4	5	6	7	8	9	10	11

SATURDAY

Goal	12	1	2	3	4	5	6	7	8	9	10	11	12	1	2	3	4	5	6	7	8	9	10	11
Actual	12	1	2	3	4	5	6	7	8	9	10	11	12	1	2	3	4	5	6	7	8	9	10	11

SUNDAY

Goal	12	1	2	3	4	5	6	7	8	9	10	11	12	1	2	3	4	5	6	7	8	9	10	11
Actual	12	1	2	3	4	5	6	7	8	9	10	11	12	1	2	3	4	5	6	7	8	9	10	11

WEEKLY *Progress*

Monday

Tuesday

Wednesday

Thursday

Friday

Saturday

Sunday

Notes

KETO *Meal* LOG BOOK

	BREAKFAST	LUNCH	DINNER	SNACKS
MONDAY				
TUESDAY				
WEDNESDAY				
THURSDAY				
FRIDAY				
SATURDAY				
SUNDAY				

MY PROGRESS *Tracker*

SLEEP TRACKER:

DATE _____

 RISE: _____   BEDTIME: _____   SLEEP (HRS): _____

NOTES FOR THE DAY

_____

_____

_____

IN A STATE OF KETOSIS?

YES   NO   UNSURE

WATER INTAKE TRACKER

EXERCISE / WORKOUT ROUTINE

DAILY ENERGY LEVEL		
HIGH	**MEDIUM**	**LOW**

BREAKFAST

FAT: CARBS: PROTEIN: CALORIES:

LUNCH

FAT: CARBS: PROTEIN: CALORIES:

DINNER

FAT: CARBS: PROTEIN: CALORIES:

SNACKS

FAT: CARBS: PROTEIN: CALORIES:

TOP 6 PRIORITIES OF THE DAY

END OF THE DAY TOTAL OVERVIEW

CARBS	FAT	PROTEIN	CALORIES

WEIGHT LOSS *Tracker*

MONTHLY GOAL

DATE:

	BUST				
	WAIST				
	HIPS				
	BICEP				
	THIGH				
	CALF				
	WEIGHT				

TOTAL WEIGHT LOSS >>

MONTHLY PROGRESS *Tracker*

JAN	FEB	MAR	APR	MAY	JUN	JUL	AUG	SEP	OCT	NOV	DEC

MON	TUE	WED	THU	FRI	SAT	SUN

WEIGHT LOSS MILESTONE TRACKER

CHEAT DAY TRACKER

WEEKLY DIET SUCCESS TRACKER & NOTES

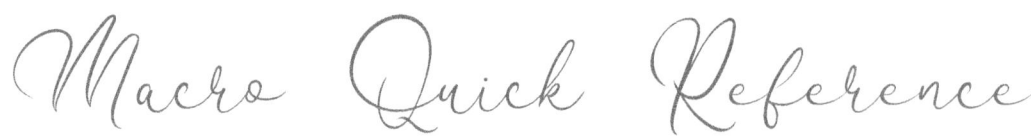

Macro Quick Reference

MACRO TRACKER

QTY	TYPE	PROTEIN	FAT	CARBS	CALS	NOTES

INTERMITTENT *Fasting Log*

WEEK OF: _____

	START TIME	END TIME	TOTAL FAST HRS
M	:	:	:
T	:	:	:
W	:	:	:
T	:	:	:
F	:	:	:
S	:	:	:
S	:	:	:

WEEK OF: _____

	START TIME	END TIME	TOTAL FAST HRS
M	:	:	:
T	:	:	:
W	:	:	:
T	:	:	:
F	:	:	:
S	:	:	:
S	:	:	:

WEEK OF: _____

	START TIME	END TIME	TOTAL FAST HRS
M	:	:	:
T	:	:	:
W	:	:	:
T	:	:	:
F	:	:	:
S	:	:	:
S	:	:	:

WEEK OF: _____

	START TIME	END TIME	TOTAL FAST HRS
M	:	:	:
T	:	:	:
W	:	:	:
T	:	:	:
F	:	:	:
S	:	:	:
S	:	:	:

WEEK OF: _____

	START TIME	END TIME	TOTAL FAST HRS
M	:	:	:
T	:	:	:
W	:	:	:
T	:	:	:
F	:	:	:
S	:	:	:
S	:	:	:

WEEK OF: _____

	START TIME	END TIME	TOTAL FAST HRS
M	:	:	:
T	:	:	:
W	:	:	:
T	:	:	:
F	:	:	:
S	:	:	:
S	:	:	:

MILESTONES & ACCOMPLISHMENTS

NOTES & REFLECTIONS

GOALS & *Accomplishments*

Month JAN FEB MAR APR MAY JUN JUL AUG SEP OCT NOV DEC

THIS MONTH'S **GOALS**

ACTION PLAN

M T W T F S S

☐☐☐☐☐☐☐
☐☐☐☐☐☐☐
☐☐☐☐☐☐☐
☐☐☐☐☐☐☐
☐☐☐☐☐☐☐

NOTES:

WEEKLY GOALS

M
T
W
T
F
S
S

THOUGHTS

MEALS:	BREAKFAST	LUNCH	DINNER	SNACKS
M				
T				
W				
T				
F				
S				
S				

Low Carb Grocery Ideas

FRESH PRODUCE

☐ Asparagus	☐ Cauliflower	☐ Onions
☐ Avocado	☐ Celery	☐ Radishes
☐ Bell Peppers	☐ Cucumber	☐ Salad Mix
☐ Berries	☐ Eggplant	☐ Squash
☐ Broccoli	☐ Fennel	☐ Tomatoes
☐ Brussel Sprouts	☐ Garlic	☐ Bok Choi
☐ Cabbage	☐ Green Beans	☐ Chives
☐ Carrots	☐ Mushrooms	☐ Spinach

MEAT AND SEAFOOD

☐ Bacon	☐ Lamb	☐ Fish
☐ Beef	☐ Pork	☐ Crab
☐ Bison	☐ Rotisserie Chicken	☐ Lobster
☐ Chicken	☐ Sausage	☐ Scallops
☐ Deli meat	☐ Turkey	☐ Shrimp
☐ Ground Beef / Ground Turkey	☐ Oyster	☐ Mussels

DAIRY PRODUCTS

☐ Butter	☐ Eggs	☐ Sour Cream
☐ Cheese	☐ Greek Yogurt, full fat	☐ Ghee
☐ Cream Cheese	☐ Heavy Whipping Cream	☐ Mayo

PANTRY ITEMS

☐ Avocado oil	☐ Tea/Coffee	☐ Moon Cheese
☐ Beef Jerky	☐ Pork Rinds	☐ Low Carb Protein Bars
☐ Bone Broth	☐ Mayonnaise	☐ All Natural Peanut Butter
☐ Tuna, Salmon (canned)	☐ Low Carb Salad Dressing	☐ Stevia
☐ Coconut Butter	☐ Olive oil, extra virgin	☐ Almonds
☐ Coconut Oil	☐ Olives	☐ Spices
☐ Almond Milk	☐ Sweeteners	☐ Almond Flour

FROZEN / OTHER

Low Carb Shopping List

FRESH PRODUCE

MEAT AND SEAFOOD

DAIRY PRODUCTS

PANTRY ITEMS

FROZEN / OTHER

Keto Friendly Foods

KETO FRIENDLY FOODS	NET CARBS	PROTEINS	FAT

FOODS TO EAT IN MODERATION	NET CARBS	PROTEINS	FAT

STAYING *On Track*

MY WEIGHT LOSS DIARY:

WATER TRACKER

LOW CARB SNACKS

NOTES & REMINDERS

DOODLE MY MOOD

BREAKFAST IDEAS

LUNCH IDEAS

DINNER IDEAS

STAYING *On Track*

MY WEIGHT LOSS DIARY:

_____

_____

_____

_____

WATER TRACKER

NOTES & REMINDERS

DOODLE MY MOOD

LOW CARB SNACKS

BREAKFAST IDEAS

LUNCH IDEAS

DINNER IDEAS

STAYING *On Track*

MY WEIGHT LOSS DIARY:

WATER TRACKER

LOW CARB SNACKS

NOTES & REMINDERS

DOODLE MY MOOD

BREAKFAST IDEAS

LUNCH IDEAS

DINNER IDEAS

STAYING *On Track*

MY WEIGHT LOSS DIARY:

_____

_____

_____

_____

WATER TRACKER

NOTES & REMINDERS

DOODLE MY MOOD

LOW CARB SNACKS

BREAKFAST IDEAS

LUNCH IDEAS

DINNER IDEAS

STAYING *On Track*

MY WEIGHT LOSS DIARY:

WATER TRACKER

NOTES & REMINDERS

DOODLE MY MOOD

LOW CARB SNACKS

BREAKFAST IDEAS

LUNCH IDEAS

DINNER IDEAS

STAYING *On Track*

MY WEIGHT LOSS DIARY:

_____
_____
_____
_____

WATER TRACKER

NOTES & REMINDERS

DOODLE MY MOOD

LOW CARB SNACKS

BREAKFAST IDEAS

LUNCH IDEAS

DINNER IDEAS

STAYING *On Track*

MY WEIGHT LOSS DIARY:

WATER TRACKER

LOW CARB SNACKS

NOTES & REMINDERS

DOODLE MY MOOD

BREAKFAST IDEAS

LUNCH IDEAS

DINNER IDEAS

MEAL *Planner*

WEEK OF

GROCERY LIST

- [ ]
- [ ]
- [ ]
- [ ]
- [ ]
- [ ]
- [ ]
- [ ]
- [ ]
- [ ]
- [ ]
- [ ]
- [ ]
- [ ]
- [ ]
- [ ]

MON

TUES

WED

THUR

FRI

SAT

SUN

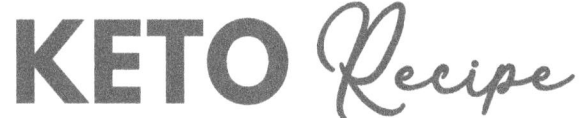

KETO *Recipe*

RECIPE NAME:

Keto	Low Carb	Paleo	Vegetarian	Vegan	Dairy Free	Gluten Free
☐	☐	☐	☐	☐	☐	☐

QTY	INGREDIENTS	RECIPE INSTRUCTIONS

NOTES & RECIPE REVIEW

Serves	
Prep Time	
Cook Time	
Tools	
Temp	

Total	Carbs	Fat	Protein	Cals

DAILY FOOD *Tracker*

FOOD TRACKER

MEAL/SNACK	NET CARBS	FAT	CAL	PROTEIN
DAILY GOAL:				
TOTAL:				

NOTES & MEAL IDEAS

FITNESS TRACKER

Type		Notes
Time		
Avg HR		
Max HR		
Reps		
Cals		

DAILY OVERVIEW

Sleep		Notes		On Track
Water Intake				
Steps Taken				
Active Mins				Goal Met
Active Hours				
Cals Burned				

DAILY FOOD *Tracker*

FOOD TRACKER

MEAL/SNACK	NET CARBS	FAT	CAL	PROTEIN

DAILY GOAL:

TOTAL:

NOTES & MEAL IDEAS

FITNESS TRACKER

Type		Notes
Time		
Avg HR		
Max HR		
Reps		
Cals		

DAILY OVERVIEW

Sleep		Notes	On Track
Water Intake			
Steps Taken			
Active Mins			Goal Met
Active Hours			
Cals Burned			

DAILY FOOD *Tracker*

FOOD TRACKER

MEAL/SNACK	NET CARBS	FAT	CAL	PROTEIN
DAILY GOAL:				
TOTAL:				

NOTES & MEAL IDEAS

FITNESS TRACKER

		Notes
Type		
Time		
Avg HR		
Max HR		
Reps		
Cals		

DAILY OVERVIEW

		Notes		
Sleep			On Track	
Water Intake				
Steps Taken				
Active Mins			Goal Met	
Active Hours				
Cals Burned				

DAILY FOOD *Tracker*

FOOD TRACKER

MEAL/SNACK	NET CARBS	FAT	CAL	PROTEIN

DAILY GOAL:				
TOTAL:				

NOTES & MEAL IDEAS

FITNESS TRACKER

		Notes
Type		
Time		
Avg HR		
Max HR		
Reps		
Cals		

DAILY OVERVIEW

		Notes		On Track
Sleep				
Water Intake				
Steps Taken				
Active Mins				Goal Met
Active Hours				
Cals Burned				

DAILY FOOD *Tracker*

FOOD TRACKER

MEAL/SNACK	NET CARBS	FAT	CAL	PROTEIN
DAILY GOAL:				
TOTAL:				

NOTES & MEAL IDEAS

FITNESS TRACKER

		Notes
Type		
Time		
Avg HR		
Max HR		
Reps		
Cals		

DAILY OVERVIEW

		Notes		
Sleep			On Track	
Water Intake				
Steps Taken				
Active Mins			Goal Met	
Active Hours				
Cals Burned				

DAILY FOOD *Tracker*

FOOD TRACKER

MEAL/SNACK	NET CARBS	FAT	CAL	PROTEIN
DAILY GOAL:				
TOTAL:				

NOTES & MEAL IDEAS

FITNESS TRACKER

		Notes
Type		
Time		
Avg HR		
Max HR		
Reps		
Cals		

DAILY OVERVIEW

		Notes		On Track
Sleep				
Water Intake				☐
Steps Taken				
Active Mins				Goal Met
Active Hours				☐
Cals Burned				

DAILY FOOD *Tracker*

FOOD TRACKER

MEAL/SNACK	NET CARBS	FAT	CAL	PROTEIN
DAILY GOAL:				
TOTAL:				

NOTES & MEAL IDEAS

FITNESS TRACKER

		Notes
Type		
Time		
Avg HR		
Max HR		
Reps		
Cals		

DAILY OVERVIEW

		Notes		
Sleep			On Track	
Water Intake				
Steps Taken				
Active Mins			Goal Met	
Active Hours				
Cals Burned				

KETO GO TO *Meals*

BREAKFAST	LUNCH	DINNER	SNACKS

BREAKFAST	LUNCH	DINNER	SNACKS

BREAKFAST	LUNCH	DINNER	SNACKS

BREAKFAST	LUNCH	DINNER	SNACKS

BREAKFAST	LUNCH	DINNER	SNACKS

BREAKFAST	LUNCH	DINNER	SNACKS

BREAKFAST	LUNCH	DINNER	SNACKS

12 WEEK *Keto Meal Tracker*

12 Week Keto Challenge

MONTH	JAN	FEB	MAR	APR	MAY	JUN	JUL	AUG	SEP	OCT	NOV	DEC
WEEK	01	02	03	04	05	06	07	08	09	10	11	12

	BREAKFAST	LUNCH	DINNER	SNACKS
M				
T				
W				
T				
F				
S				
S				

GROCERY SHOPPING LIST / RECIPE INGREDIENTS

Weekly Meal Planner

Week of: _____

	Breakfast	Lunch	Dinner	Snack	Other
Monday	TOTAL Carbs Fat Protein Cals	TOTAL Carbs Fat Protein Cals	TOTAL Carbs Fat Protein Cals	TOTAL Carbs Fat Protein Cals	TOTAL Carbs Fat Protein Cals
Tuesday	TOTAL Carbs Fat Protein Cals	TOTAL Carbs Fat Protein Cals	TOTAL Carbs Fat Protein Cals	TOTAL Carbs Fat Protein Cals	TOTAL Carbs Fat Protein Cals
Wednesday	TOTAL Carbs Fat Protein Cals	TOTAL Carbs Fat Protein Cals	TOTAL Carbs Fat Protein Cals	TOTAL Carbs Fat Protein Cals	TOTAL Carbs Fat Protein Cals
Thursday	TOTAL Carbs Fat Protein Cals	TOTAL Carbs Fat Protein Cals	TOTAL Carbs Fat Protein Cals	TOTAL Carbs Fat Protein Cals	TOTAL Carbs Fat Protein Cals
Friday	TOTAL Carbs Fat Protein Cals	TOTAL Carbs Fat Protein Cals	TOTAL Carbs Fat Protein Cals	TOTAL Carbs Fat Protein Cals	TOTAL Carbs Fat Protein Cals
Saturday	TOTAL Carbs Fat Protein Cals	TOTAL Carbs Fat Protein Cals	TOTAL Carbs Fat Protein Cals	TOTAL Carbs Fat Protein Cals	TOTAL Carbs Fat Protein Cals
Sunday	TOTAL Carbs Fat Protein Cals	TOTAL Carbs Fat Protein Cals	TOTAL Carbs Fat Protein Cals	TOTAL Carbs Fat Protein Cals	TOTAL Carbs Fat Protein Cals

WEIGHT LOSS *Journal*

MONDAY

TUESDAY

WEDNESDAY

THURSDAY

FRIDAY

SATURDAY

SUNDAY

WEEK OF:

DATE	WEIGHT LOSS ACTION PLAN

NOTES

MY WEIGHT LOSS *Routine*

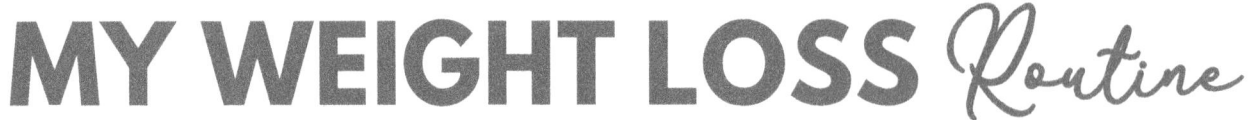

CREATING A ROUTINE FOR SUCCESS

WEIGHT LOSS SUCCESS: HABIT & ROUTINE TRACKER	
DRINK LOTS OF WATER TODAY	**TRACK TOTAL CARB INTAKE**

COMPLETE TOP 3 GOALS OF THE DAY

1
2
3

PLAN MY MEALS FOR THE DAY:

BREAKFAST	LUNCH	DINNER

DAILY TRACKER & TO DO LIST	ACCOMPLISHMENTS

NOTES

WEEKLY *Fasting Tracker*

Week Of: _____

MONDAY

Goal	12	1	2	3	4	5	6	7	8	9	10	11	12	1	2	3	4	5	6	7	8	9	10	11
Actual	12	1	2	3	4	5	6	7	8	9	10	11	12	1	2	3	4	5	6	7	8	9	10	11

TUESDAY

Goal	12	1	2	3	4	5	6	7	8	9	10	11	12	1	2	3	4	5	6	7	8	9	10	11
Actual	12	1	2	3	4	5	6	7	8	9	10	11	12	1	2	3	4	5	6	7	8	9	10	11

WEDNESDAY

Goal	12	1	2	3	4	5	6	7	8	9	10	11	12	1	2	3	4	5	6	7	8	9	10	11
Actual	12	1	2	3	4	5	6	7	8	9	10	11	12	1	2	3	4	5	6	7	8	9	10	11

THURSDAY

Goal	12	1	2	3	4	5	6	7	8	9	10	11	12	1	2	3	4	5	6	7	8	9	10	11
Actual	12	1	2	3	4	5	6	7	8	9	10	11	12	1	2	3	4	5	6	7	8	9	10	11

FRIDAY

Goal	12	1	2	3	4	5	6	7	8	9	10	11	12	1	2	3	4	5	6	7	8	9	10	11
Actual	12	1	2	3	4	5	6	7	8	9	10	11	12	1	2	3	4	5	6	7	8	9	10	11

SATURDAY

Goal	12	1	2	3	4	5	6	7	8	9	10	11	12	1	2	3	4	5	6	7	8	9	10	11
Actual	12	1	2	3	4	5	6	7	8	9	10	11	12	1	2	3	4	5	6	7	8	9	10	11

SUNDAY

Goal	12	1	2	3	4	5	6	7	8	9	10	11	12	1	2	3	4	5	6	7	8	9	10	11
Actual	12	1	2	3	4	5	6	7	8	9	10	11	12	1	2	3	4	5	6	7	8	9	10	11

WEEKLY *Progress*

Monday

Tuesday

Wednesday

Thursday

Friday

Saturday

Sunday

Notes

KETO *Meal* LOG BOOK

	BREAKFAST	LUNCH	DINNER	SNACKS
MONDAY				
TUESDAY				
WEDNESDAY				
THURSDAY				
FRIDAY				
SATURDAY				
SUNDAY				

MY PROGRESS *Tracker*

SLEEP TRACKER:

DATE

RISE: BEDTIME: SLEEP (HRS):

NOTES FOR THE DAY

IN A STATE OF KETOSIS?

YES   NO   UNSURE

WATER INTAKE TRACKER

EXERCISE / WORKOUT ROUTINE

DAILY ENERGY LEVEL		
HIGH	**MEDIUM**	**LOW**

BREAKFAST

FAT: CARBS: PROTEIN: CALORIES:

LUNCH

FAT: CARBS: PROTEIN: CALORIES:

DINNER

FAT: CARBS: PROTEIN: CALORIES:

SNACKS

FAT: CARBS: PROTEIN: CALORIES:

TOP 6 PRIORITIES OF THE DAY

END OF THE DAY TOTAL OVERVIEW

CARBS	FAT	PROTEIN	CALORIES

Macro Quick Reference

MACRO TRACKER

QTY	TYPE	PROTEIN	FAT	CARBS	CALS	NOTES

INTERMITTENT *Fasting Log*

WEEK OF:

	START TIME	END TIME	TOTAL FAST HRS
M	:	:	:
T	:	:	:
W	:	:	:
T	:	:	:
F	:	:	:
S	:	:	:
S	:	:	:

WEEK OF:

	START TIME	END TIME	TOTAL FAST HRS
M	:	:	:
T	:	:	:
W	:	:	:
T	:	:	:
F	:	:	:
S	:	:	:
S	:	:	:

WEEK OF:

	START TIME	END TIME	TOTAL FAST HRS
M	:	:	:
T	:	:	:
W	:	:	:
T	:	:	:
F	:	:	:
S	:	:	:
S	:	:	:

WEEK OF:

	START TIME	END TIME	TOTAL FAST HRS
M	:	:	:
T	:	:	:
W	:	:	:
T	:	:	:
F	:	:	:
S	:	:	:
S	:	:	:

WEEK OF:

	START TIME	END TIME	TOTAL FAST HRS
M	:	:	:
T	:	:	:
W	:	:	:
T	:	:	:
F	:	:	:
S	:	:	:
S	:	:	:

WEEK OF:

	START TIME	END TIME	TOTAL FAST HRS
M	:	:	:
T	:	:	:
W	:	:	:
T	:	:	:
F	:	:	:
S	:	:	:
S	:	:	:

MILESTONES & ACCOMPLISHMENTS

NOTES & REFLECTIONS

GOALS & *Accomplishments*

THIS MONTH'S **GOALS**

ACTION PLAN

M T W T F S S

☐☐☐☐☐☐☐
☐☐☐☐☐☐☐
☐☐☐☐☐☐☐
☐☐☐☐☐☐☐
☐☐☐☐☐☐☐

NOTES:

WEEKLY GOALS

M

T

W

T

F

S

S

THOUGHTS

MEALS:	BREAKFAST	LUNCH	DINNER	SNACKS
M				
T				
W				
T				
F				
S				
S				

Low Carb Shopping List

FRESH PRODUCE

MEAT AND SEAFOOD

DAIRY PRODUCTS

PANTRY ITEMS

FROZEN / OTHER

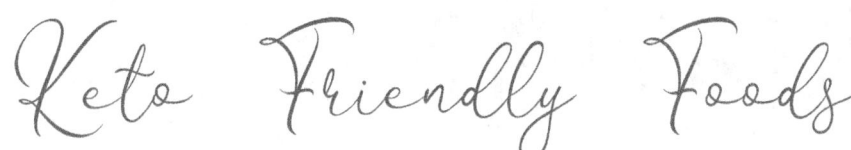

Keto Friendly Foods

KETO FRIENDLY FOODS	NET CARBS	PROTEINS	FAT

FOODS TO EAT IN MODERATION	NET CARBS	PROTEINS	FAT

STAYING *On Track*

MY WEIGHT LOSS DIARY:

WATER TRACKER

LOW CARB SNACKS

NOTES & REMINDERS

DOODLE MY MOOD

BREAKFAST IDEAS

LUNCH IDEAS

DINNER IDEAS

STAYING *On Track*

MY WEIGHT LOSS DIARY:

_____

_____

_____

_____

WATER TRACKER

○ ○ ○ ○ ○ ○ ○ ○

LOW CARB SNACKS

NOTES & REMINDERS

DOODLE MY MOOD

BREAKFAST IDEAS

LUNCH IDEAS

DINNER IDEAS

STAYING *On Track*

MY WEIGHT LOSS DIARY:

WATER TRACKER

NOTES & REMINDERS

DOODLE MY MOOD

LOW CARB SNACKS

BREAKFAST IDEAS

LUNCH IDEAS

DINNER IDEAS

STAYING *On Track*

MY WEIGHT LOSS DIARY:

_____
_____
_____
_____

WATER TRACKER

NOTES & REMINDERS

DOODLE MY MOOD

LOW CARB SNACKS

BREAKFAST IDEAS

LUNCH IDEAS

DINNER IDEAS

STAYING *On Track*

MY WEIGHT LOSS DIARY:

WATER TRACKER

LOW CARB SNACKS

NOTES & REMINDERS

DOODLE MY MOOD

BREAKFAST IDEAS

LUNCH IDEAS

DINNER IDEAS

STAYING *On Track*

MY WEIGHT LOSS DIARY:

_____

_____

_____

_____

WATER TRACKER

LOW CARB SNACKS

NOTES & REMINDERS

DOODLE MY MOOD

BREAKFAST IDEAS

LUNCH IDEAS

DINNER IDEAS

STAYING *On Track*

MY WEIGHT LOSS DIARY:

WATER TRACKER

LOW CARB SNACKS

NOTES & REMINDERS

DOODLE MY MOOD

BREAKFAST IDEAS

LUNCH IDEAS

DINNER IDEAS

MEAL *Planner*

WEEK OF

GROCERY LIST

- [ ]
- [ ]
- [ ]
- [ ]
- [ ]
- [ ]
- [ ]
- [ ]
- [ ]
- [ ]
- [ ]
- [ ]
- [ ]
- [ ]
- [ ]
- [ ]
- [ ]

MON

TUES

WED

THUR

FRI

SAT

SUN

KETO *Recipe*

RECIPE NAME:

Keto	Low Carb	Paleo	Vegetarian	Vegan	Dairy Free	Gluten Free
☐	☐	☐	☐	☐	☐	☐

QTY	INGREDIENTS	RECIPE INSTRUCTIONS

NOTES & RECIPE REVIEW

	Serves
	Prep Time
	Cook Time
	Tools
	Temp

Total	Carbs	Fat	Protein	Cals

DAILY FOOD *Tracker*

FOOD TRACKER

MEAL/SNACK	NET CARBS	FAT	CAL	PROTEIN
DAILY GOAL:				
TOTAL:				

NOTES & MEAL IDEAS

FITNESS TRACKER

		Notes
Type		
Time		
Avg HR		
Max HR		
Reps		
Cals		

DAILY OVERVIEW

		Notes		On Track
Sleep				
Water Intake				
Steps Taken				
Active Mins				Goal Met
Active Hours				
Cals Burned				

DAILY FOOD *Tracker*

FOOD TRACKER

MEAL/SNACK	NET CARBS	FAT	CAL	PROTEIN
DAILY GOAL:				
TOTAL:				

NOTES & MEAL IDEAS

FITNESS TRACKER

		Notes
Type		
Time		
Avg HR		
Max HR		
Reps		
Cals		

DAILY OVERVIEW

		Notes		On Track
Sleep				
Water Intake				
Steps Taken				
Active Mins				Goal Met
Active Hours				
Cals Burned				

DAILY FOOD *Tracker*

FOOD TRACKER

MEAL/SNACK	NET CARBS	FAT	CAL	PROTEIN
DAILY GOAL:				
TOTAL:				

NOTES & MEAL IDEAS

FITNESS TRACKER

		Notes
Type		
Time		
Avg HR		
Max HR		
Reps		
Cals		

DAILY OVERVIEW

		Notes		On Track
Sleep				
Water Intake				☐
Steps Taken				
Active Mins				Goal Met
Active Hours				
Cals Burned				☐

DAILY FOOD *Tracker*

FOOD TRACKER

MEAL/SNACK	NET CARBS	FAT	CAL	PROTEIN

DAILY GOAL:

TOTAL:

NOTES & MEAL IDEAS

FITNESS TRACKER

		Notes
Type		
Time		
Avg HR		
Max HR		
Reps		
Cals		

DAILY OVERVIEW

		Notes		On Track
Sleep				
Water Intake				
Steps Taken				
Active Mins				Goal Met
Active Hours				
Cals Burned				

DAILY FOOD *Tracker*

FOOD TRACKER

MEAL/SNACK	NET CARBS	FAT	CAL	PROTEIN

	NET CARBS	FAT	CAL	PROTEIN
DAILY GOAL:				
TOTAL:				

NOTES & MEAL IDEAS

FITNESS TRACKER

		Notes
Type		
Time		
Avg HR		
Max HR		
Reps		
Cals		

DAILY OVERVIEW

		Notes		On Track
Sleep				
Water Intake				
Steps Taken				
Active Mins				Goal Met
Active Hours				
Cals Burned				

DAILY FOOD *Tracker*

FOOD TRACKER

MEAL/SNACK	NET CARBS	FAT	CAL	PROTEIN
DAILY GOAL:				
TOTAL:				

NOTES & MEAL IDEAS

FITNESS TRACKER

		Notes
Type		
Time		
Avg HR		
Max HR		
Reps		
Cals		

DAILY OVERVIEW

		Notes		On Track
Sleep				
Water Intake				
Steps Taken				
Active Mins				Goal Met
Active Hours				
Cals Burned				

DAILY FOOD *Tracker*

FOOD TRACKER

MEAL/SNACK	NET CARBS	FAT	CAL	PROTEIN
DAILY GOAL:				
TOTAL:				

NOTES & MEAL IDEAS

FITNESS TRACKER

		Notes
Type		
Time		
Avg HR		
Max HR		
Reps		
Cals		

DAILY OVERVIEW

		Notes		On Track
Sleep				
Water Intake				
Steps Taken				
Active Mins				Goal Met
Active Hours				
Cals Burned				

KETO GO TO *Meals*

FAVORITE KETO FRIENDLY MEALS

BREAKFAST	LUNCH	DINNER	SNACKS
BREAKFAST	LUNCH	DINNER	SNACKS
BREAKFAST	LUNCH	DINNER	SNACKS
BREAKFAST	LUNCH	DINNER	SNACKS
BREAKFAST	LUNCH	DINNER	SNACKS
BREAKFAST	LUNCH	DINNER	SNACKS
BREAKFAST	LUNCH	DINNER	SNACKS

12 WEEK *Keto Meal Tracker*

12 Week Keto Challenge

MONTH	JAN	FEB	MAR	APR	MAY	JUN	JUL	AUG	SEP	OCT	NOV	DEC
WEEK	01	02	03	04	05	06	07	08	09	10	11	12

	BREAKFAST	LUNCH	DINNER	SNACKS
M				
T				
W				
T				
F				
S				
S				

GROCERY SHOPPING LIST / RECIPE INGREDIENTS

WEIGHT LOSS *Journal*

MONDAY

TUESDAY

WEDNESDAY

THURSDAY

FRIDAY

SATURDAY

SUNDAY

WEEK OF:

DATE	WEIGHT LOSS ACTION PLAN

NOTES

WEIGHT LOSS *Tracker*

MONTHLY GOAL

DATE:

	BUST				
	WAIST				
	HIPS				
	BICEP				
	THIGH				
	CALF				
	WEIGHT				

TOTAL WEIGHT LOSS >>

MONTHLY PROGRESS *Tracker*

JAN   FEB   MAR   APR   MAY   JUN   JUL   AUG   SEP   OCT   NOV   DEC

MON	TUE	WED	THU	FRI	SAT	SUN

WEIGHT LOSS MILESTONE TRACKER

CHEAT DAY TRACKER

WEEKLY DIET SUCCESS TRACKER & NOTES

MY WEIGHT LOSS *Routine*

CREATING A ROUTINE FOR SUCCESS

WEIGHT LOSS SUCCESS: HABIT & ROUTINE TRACKER

DRINK LOTS OF WATER TODAY	TRACK TOTAL CARB INTAKE

COMPLETE TOP 3 GOALS OF THE DAY

1

2

3

PLAN MY MEALS FOR THE DAY:

BREAKFAST	LUNCH	DINNER

DAILY TRACKER & TO DO LIST	ACCOMPLISHMENTS

NOTES

WEEKLY *Fasting Tracker*

Week Of: _____

MONDAY

Goal	12	1	2	3	4	5	6	7	8	9	10	11	12	1	2	3	4	5	6	7	8	9	10	11
Actual	12	1	2	3	4	5	6	7	8	9	10	11	12	1	2	3	4	5	6	7	8	9	10	11

TUESDAY

Goal	12	1	2	3	4	5	6	7	8	9	10	11	12	1	2	3	4	5	6	7	8	9	10	11
Actual	12	1	2	3	4	5	6	7	8	9	10	11	12	1	2	3	4	5	6	7	8	9	10	11

WEDNESDAY

Goal	12	1	2	3	4	5	6	7	8	9	10	11	12	1	2	3	4	5	6	7	8	9	10	11
Actual	12	1	2	3	4	5	6	7	8	9	10	11	12	1	2	3	4	5	6	7	8	9	10	11

THURSDAY

Goal	12	1	2	3	4	5	6	7	8	9	10	11	12	1	2	3	4	5	6	7	8	9	10	11
Actual	12	1	2	3	4	5	6	7	8	9	10	11	12	1	2	3	4	5	6	7	8	9	10	11

FRIDAY

Goal	12	1	2	3	4	5	6	7	8	9	10	11	12	1	2	3	4	5	6	7	8	9	10	11
Actual	12	1	2	3	4	5	6	7	8	9	10	11	12	1	2	3	4	5	6	7	8	9	10	11

SATURDAY

Goal	12	1	2	3	4	5	6	7	8	9	10	11	12	1	2	3	4	5	6	7	8	9	10	11
Actual	12	1	2	3	4	5	6	7	8	9	10	11	12	1	2	3	4	5	6	7	8	9	10	11

SUNDAY

Goal	12	1	2	3	4	5	6	7	8	9	10	11	12	1	2	3	4	5	6	7	8	9	10	11
Actual	12	1	2	3	4	5	6	7	8	9	10	11	12	1	2	3	4	5	6	7	8	9	10	11

KETO *Meal* LOG BOOK

	BREAKFAST	LUNCH	DINNER	SNACKS
MONDAY				
TUESDAY				
WEDNESDAY				
THURSDAY				
FRIDAY				
SATURDAY				
SUNDAY				

MY PROGRESS *Tracker*

SLEEP TRACKER:

DATE

RISE: BEDTIME: SLEEP (HRS):

NOTES FOR THE DAY

IN A STATE OF KETOSIS?

YES   NO   UNSURE

WATER INTAKE TRACKER

EXERCISE / WORKOUT ROUTINE

DAILY ENERGY LEVEL		
HIGH	**MEDIUM**	**LOW**

BREAKFAST

FAT: CARBS: PROTEIN: CALORIES:

LUNCH

FAT: CARBS: PROTEIN: CALORIES:

DINNER

FAT: CARBS: PROTEIN: CALORIES:

SNACKS

FAT: CARBS: PROTEIN: CALORIES:

TOP 6 PRIORITIES OF THE DAY

END OF THE DAY TOTAL OVERVIEW

CARBS   FAT   PROTEIN   CALORIES

Macro Quick Reference

MACRO TRACKER

QTY	TYPE	PROTEIN	FAT	CARBS	CALS	NOTES

INTERMITTENT *Fasting Log*

WEEK OF:

	START TIME	END TIME	TOTAL FAST HRS
M	:	:	:
T	:	:	:
W	:	:	:
T	:	:	:
F	:	:	:
S	:	:	:
S	:	:	:

WEEK OF:

	START TIME	END TIME	TOTAL FAST HRS
M	:	:	:
T	:	:	:
W	:	:	:
T	:	:	:
F	:	:	:
S	:	:	:
S	:	:	:

WEEK OF:

	START TIME	END TIME	TOTAL FAST HRS
M	:	:	:
T	:	:	:
W	:	:	:
T	:	:	:
F	:	:	:
S	:	:	:
S	:	:	:

WEEK OF:

	START TIME	END TIME	TOTAL FAST HRS
M	:	:	:
T	:	:	:
W	:	:	:
T	:	:	:
F	:	:	:
S	:	:	:
S	:	:	:

WEEK OF:

	START TIME	END TIME	TOTAL FAST HRS
M	:	:	:
T	:	:	:
W	:	:	:
T	:	:	:
F	:	:	:
S	:	:	:
S	:	:	:

WEEK OF:

	START TIME	END TIME	TOTAL FAST HRS
M	:	:	:
T	:	:	:
W	:	:	:
T	:	:	:
F	:	:	:
S	:	:	:
S	:	:	:

MILESTONES & ACCOMPLISHMENTS

NOTES & REFLECTIONS

GOALS & *Accomplishments*

Month | JAN FEB MAR APR MAY JUN JUL AUG SEP OCT NOV DEC

THIS MONTH'S **GOALS**

ACTION PLAN

M T W T F S S

☐ ☐ ☐ ☐ ☐ ☐ ☐
☐ ☐ ☐ ☐ ☐ ☐ ☐
☐ ☐ ☐ ☐ ☐ ☐ ☐
☐ ☐ ☐ ☐ ☐ ☐ ☐
☐ ☐ ☐ ☐ ☐ ☐ ☐

NOTES:

WEEKLY GOALS

M
T
W
T
F
S
S

THOUGHTS

MEALS:	BREAKFAST	LUNCH	DINNER	SNACKS
M				
T				
W				
T				
F				
S				
S				

Low Carb Shopping List

FRESH PRODUCE

MEAT AND SEAFOOD

DAIRY PRODUCTS

PANTRY ITEMS

FROZEN / OTHER

Keto Friendly Foods

KETO FRIENDLY FOODS	NET CARBS	PROTEINS	FAT

FOODS TO EAT IN MODERATION	NET CARBS	PROTEINS	FAT

STAYING *On Track*

MY WEIGHT LOSS DIARY:

WATER TRACKER

NOTES & REMINDERS

DOODLE MY MOOD

LOW CARB SNACKS

BREAKFAST IDEAS

LUNCH IDEAS

DINNER IDEAS

STAYING *On Track*

MY WEIGHT LOSS DIARY:

_____
_____
_____
_____

WATER TRACKER

○ ○ ○ ○ ○ ○ ○ ○

LOW CARB SNACKS

NOTES & REMINDERS

DOODLE MY MOOD

BREAKFAST IDEAS

LUNCH IDEAS

DINNER IDEAS

STAYING *On Track*

MY WEIGHT LOSS DIARY:

WATER TRACKER

NOTES & REMINDERS

DOODLE MY MOOD

LOW CARB SNACKS

BREAKFAST IDEAS

LUNCH IDEAS

DINNER IDEAS

STAYING *On Track*

MY WEIGHT LOSS DIARY:

_____

_____

_____

_____

WATER TRACKER

NOTES & REMINDERS

DOODLE MY MOOD

LOW CARB SNACKS

BREAKFAST IDEAS

LUNCH IDEAS

DINNER IDEAS

STAYING *On Track*

MY WEIGHT LOSS DIARY:

WATER TRACKER

LOW CARB SNACKS

NOTES & REMINDERS

DOODLE MY MOOD

BREAKFAST IDEAS

LUNCH IDEAS

DINNER IDEAS

STAYING *On Track*

MY WEIGHT LOSS DIARY:

_____

_____

_____

_____

WATER TRACKER

NOTES & REMINDERS

DOODLE MY MOOD

LOW CARB SNACKS

BREAKFAST IDEAS

LUNCH IDEAS

DINNER IDEAS

STAYING *On Track*

MY WEIGHT LOSS DIARY:

WATER TRACKER

LOW CARB SNACKS

NOTES & REMINDERS

DOODLE MY MOOD

BREAKFAST IDEAS

LUNCH IDEAS

DINNER IDEAS

MEAL *Planner*

GROCERY LIST

- [ ]
- [ ]
- [ ]
- [ ]
- [ ]
- [ ]
- [ ]
- [ ]
- [ ]
- [ ]
- [ ]
- [ ]
- [ ]
- [ ]
- [ ]
- [ ]
- [ ]

WEEK OF

MON

TUES

WED

THUR

FRI

SAT

SUN

KETO *Meal* LOG BOOK

	BREAKFAST	LUNCH	DINNER	SNACKS
MONDAY				
TUESDAY				
WEDNESDAY				
THURSDAY				
FRIDAY				
SATURDAY				
SUNDAY				

WEEKLY *Fasting Tracker*

Week Of: _____

MONDAY

Goal	12	1	2	3	4	5	6	7	8	9	10	11	12	1	2	3	4	5	6	7	8	9	10	11
Actual	12	1	2	3	4	5	6	7	8	9	10	11	12	1	2	3	4	5	6	7	8	9	10	11

TUESDAY

Goal	12	1	2	3	4	5	6	7	8	9	10	11	12	1	2	3	4	5	6	7	8	9	10	11
Actual	12	1	2	3	4	5	6	7	8	9	10	11	12	1	2	3	4	5	6	7	8	9	10	11

WEDNESDAY

Goal	12	1	2	3	4	5	6	7	8	9	10	11	12	1	2	3	4	5	6	7	8	9	10	11
Actual	12	1	2	3	4	5	6	7	8	9	10	11	12	1	2	3	4	5	6	7	8	9	10	11

THURSDAY

Goal	12	1	2	3	4	5	6	7	8	9	10	11	12	1	2	3	4	5	6	7	8	9	10	11
Actual	12	1	2	3	4	5	6	7	8	9	10	11	12	1	2	3	4	5	6	7	8	9	10	11

FRIDAY

Goal	12	1	2	3	4	5	6	7	8	9	10	11	12	1	2	3	4	5	6	7	8	9	10	11
Actual	12	1	2	3	4	5	6	7	8	9	10	11	12	1	2	3	4	5	6	7	8	9	10	11

SATURDAY

Goal	12	1	2	3	4	5	6	7	8	9	10	11	12	1	2	3	4	5	6	7	8	9	10	11
Actual	12	1	2	3	4	5	6	7	8	9	10	11	12	1	2	3	4	5	6	7	8	9	10	11

SUNDAY

Goal	12	1	2	3	4	5	6	7	8	9	10	11	12	1	2	3	4	5	6	7	8	9	10	11
Actual	12	1	2	3	4	5	6	7	8	9	10	11	12	1	2	3	4	5	6	7	8	9	10	11

Weekly Meal Planner

Week of: _____

	Breakfast	Lunch	Dinner	Snack	Other
Monday	TOTAL Carbs Fat Protein Cals	TOTAL Carbs Fat Protein Cals	TOTAL Carbs Fat Protein Cals	TOTAL Carbs Fat Protein Cals	TOTAL Carbs Fat Protein Cals
Tuesday	TOTAL Carbs Fat Protein Cals	TOTAL Carbs Fat Protein Cals	TOTAL Carbs Fat Protein Cals	TOTAL Carbs Fat Protein Cals	TOTAL Carbs Fat Protein Cals
Wednesday	TOTAL Carbs Fat Protein Cals	TOTAL Carbs Fat Protein Cals	TOTAL Carbs Fat Protein Cals	TOTAL Carbs Fat Protein Cals	TOTAL Carbs Fat Protein Cals
Thursday	TOTAL Carbs Fat Protein Cals	TOTAL Carbs Fat Protein Cals	TOTAL Carbs Fat Protein Cals	TOTAL Carbs Fat Protein Cals	TOTAL Carbs Fat Protein Cals
Friday	TOTAL Carbs Fat Protein Cals	TOTAL Carbs Fat Protein Cals	TOTAL Carbs Fat Protein Cals	TOTAL Carbs Fat Protein Cals	TOTAL Carbs Fat Protein Cals
Saturday	TOTAL Carbs Fat Protein Cals	TOTAL Carbs Fat Protein Cals	TOTAL Carbs Fat Protein Cals	TOTAL Carbs Fat Protein Cals	TOTAL Carbs Fat Protein Cals
Sunday	TOTAL Carbs Fat Protein Cals	TOTAL Carbs Fat Protein Cals	TOTAL Carbs Fat Protein Cals	TOTAL Carbs Fat Protein Cals	TOTAL Carbs Fat Protein Cals

WEIGHT LOSS *Journal*

MONDAY

TUESDAY

WEDNESDAY

THURSDAY

FRIDAY

SATURDAY

SUNDAY

WEEK OF:

DATE	WEIGHT LOSS ACTION PLAN

NOTES

WEIGHT LOSS *Tracker*

MONTHLY GOAL

DATE:

BUST				
WAIST				
HIPS				
BICEP				
THIGH				
CALF				
WEIGHT				

TOTAL WEIGHT LOSS >>